Atherosclerosis Pathogenesis and Microvascular Dysfunction

T0172134

Axel Haverich · Erin Colleen Boyle

Atherosclerosis Pathogenesis and Microvascular Dysfunction

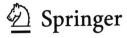 Springer

Axel Haverich
Hannover Medical School
Hannover, Niedersachsen, Germany

Erin Colleen Boyle
Hannover Medical School
Hannover, Niedersachsen, Germany

ISBN 978-3-030-20247-7   ISBN 978-3-030-20245-3   (eBook)
https://doi.org/10.1007/978-3-030-20245-3

This Springer imprint is published by the registered company Springer Nature Switzerland AG
The registered company address is: Gewerbestrasse 11, 6330 Cham, Switzerland

To my patients and colleagues
Axel Haverich

To Orla and Kilian Graßl
Erin Colleen Boyle

Preface

Based on surgical observations, I've remained critical about many of the hypotheses regarding the pathogenesis of atherosclerosis, since two important paradigms appear to be incorrect. First, atherosclerosis is not a generalized disease as defined segments of the arterial tree in humans are nearly always disease-free. Second, disease is not instigated in the endothelium of the parent vessel. Growing evidence and my observations support an "outside-in" initiation and progression of atherosclerosis development whereby vascular inflammation is initiated in the adventitia and is propagated inward toward the intima. Cardiovascular surgeons from around the world would support this.

These observations led me on a 6-year journey of research via the Internet. Very soon, though, other sources like international libraries and historic bookshops were involved providing me with remote articles and "ancient" books from the nineteenth and early twentieth centuries. I drew upon these to form the picture of the pathogenesis of atherosclerosis presented in this book. Relating my theory of atherosclerosis development over coffee one morning in Bad Nauheim, my mentor, the former director of the Max Planck Institute for Heart and Lung Research, Wolfgang Schaper, smiling broadly said, "I've worked my whole life on this topic and you've explained the whole thing in 10 minutes!" Encouraged, I next did what you always should do—I listened to an old friend, Davor Solter, a Croatian stem cell researcher and also a former Max Planck Director. When I approached him with my ideas, he immediately suggested that I compile all my findings in a book. I desperately resisted, referring to the tremendous clinical burden, being head of a busy cardiothoracic, vascular, and transplant unit. However, it would have been impossible to provide sufficient insight into the topic for the reader by an original article, a review article, or a historic note. Most surgical friends remained skeptical, only Gerd Walterbusch, my Doktorvater, surgical mentor, and long-time close friend remained a critical advisor, emphasizing the role of the lymphatic system in atherosclerosis.

The ideas put forth in this book are important for our research on primary and secondary prevention of atherosclerosis, for our trajectories in clinical diagnostics and therapy development, and finally for the patients and their families affected by this highly prevalent and deadly disease. Therefore, with the help and enthusiasm of Erin Boyle, I finally gave in and we've worked together on translating these ideas into a book. I am indeed very grateful to her because without her help in writing and completing the literature research, the book would not have been finalized until my retirement. Explanation of the molecular mechanisms involved in vasa vasorum dysfunction and protection, especially in Chap. 6, goes back primarily to Erin's research. And finally, Erin and I would like to thank Birgit Lüttig for her editorial assistance in completing this project and Daniela Martens for help with the illustrations.

Hannover, Germany   Axel Haverich
February 2019

Contents

Chapter 1
Introduction

1.1 The Known Unknowns of Atherosclerosis

"There are known knowns. There are things we know that we know. There are known unknowns. That is to say, there are things that we now know we don't know. But there are also unknown unknowns. There are things we do not know we don't know." (Donald Rumsfeld 2002) [1]

The large arteries of the human body—also named conduit arteries—can be considered as an organ by itself. They differ from the smaller distribution arteries considerably in that they:

(1) Exhibit elastic properties to maintain an adequate mean blood pressure for organ perfusion, possessing a considerable amount of collagen and elastic fibers that provide the Windkessel function to dampen the pulsatility of left ventricular pressure.

(2) Unlike distribution arteries, which are more muscular in wall construction, they possess their own vascular supply, including arterial and venous vasa vasorum. These microvessels assure adequate blood supply and drainage to provide oxygen supply and nutrients to the vessel wall.

(3) In their highly vascularized adventitial layer, these large arteries also contain lymphatic microvessels which participate in immunological functions and maintain interstitial fluid balance while also draining the vessel wall of waste and other metabolic products.

Arteriosclerosis is the general term describing a number of disorders involving the stiffening or hardening of arteries, some resulting in atheroma formation, others not. Felix Jacob Marchand from Leipzig coined the term atherosclerosis in 1904 [2], and in doing so separated the sclerotic changes seen in large conduit arteries from the phenomena of other forms of arteriosclerosis, which can also affect smaller distribution arteries and are usually linked to chronic inflammatory

© Springer Nature Switzerland AG 2019
A. Haverich and E. C. Boyle, *Atherosclerosis Pathogenesis and Microvascular Dysfunction*, https://doi.org/10.1007/978-3-030-20245-3_1

diseases (rheumatic conditions, diabetes, renal failure, and specific infectious diseases like typhoid fever). In this book, we will focus on atherosclerosis—the most serious and clinically relevant form of arteriosclerosis that is characterized by the progressive buildup of plaque inside artery walls commonly leading to restricted blood flow which then may cause clinical symptoms. Atherosclerotic cardiovascular and cerebrovascular diseases are the leading causes of death not only in developed countries. Primarily due to an increase in atherosclerosis, it is projected that by 2030, deaths due to cardiovascular and cerebrovascular diseases will increase to 22 million per year [3]. Yet astonishingly, despite decades of research, the pathomechanisms of disease development are still not known.

"The problem of the origin and development of arteriosclerosis has been attacked by many investigators in a great many ways, but in spite of all efforts, an altogether satisfactory solution has not been found." (William Ophüls 1921) [4]

"The causation of arteriosclerosis is not understood, and innumerable empirical efforts to reproduce the disease experimentally have been futile." (Winternitz et al. 1938) [5]

"Atherosclerosis has been of interest for more than a century and the characteristic morphologic changes are well known; yet its etiology remains obscure." (Oscar Creech 1957) [6]

"At the present time it does not seem possible to bring together all the available information into a unifying concept which will explain the cause and development of the lesions." (John E. French 1966) [7]

"The causes of arteriosclerosis are still largely unknown." (Hauss et al. 1990) [8]

"Despite the fact that millions of dollars have been spent over the last 50 years on atherosclerosis research, little is known about the development of early human atherosclerosis." (Nakashima et al. 2008) [9]

"The exact cause of atherosclerosis isn't known." (National Institute of Health, accessed Sept. 18, 2018) [10]

During a professional lifetime, angiologists, radiologists, and cardiovascular surgeons see thousands of images of the arterial vascular tree in subjects with or without atherosclerosis. While cardiologists focus on coronary blood vessels, angiologists look at those responsible for peripheral circulation. Both will describe their findings based on contrast injections which illuminate only the luminal contours of blood vessels. Surgeons and pathologists, by contrast, have the opportunity to visualize both luminal aspects as well as characteristics of the vessel wall and surrounding tissue. Only recently have three-dimensional imaging procedures allowed for in vivo assessment of arterial wall structures by, for example, optical coherence tomography or magnetic resonance imaging studies [11].

Technical advances in computed tomography (CT) technology, including significantly lower radiation hazards, have increased the number of films, where indeed a detailed comparison between the left and right aortoiliac–femoral axis has become common practice. Looking at such images in patients with calcifying atherosclerosis, a surprising **symmetry of bilateral calcification** can be seen in many subjects (Fig. 1.1). At the same time, a surprising degree of **asymmetry** is found looking at calcified regions in **cross-sectional images**. Often, less than half of the circular wall is affected, a picture well known from histological, cross-sectional slides of atherosclerotic arteries and well known from textbooks. Here, major segments of the arterial circumference are actually free from

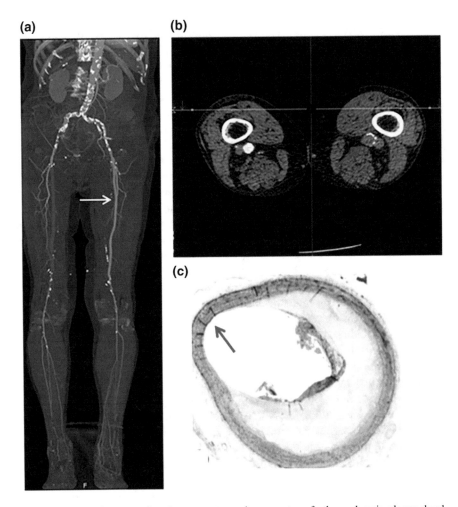

Fig. 1.1 Images demonstrating the symmetry and asymmetry of atherosclerosis plaque development in humans. **a** Maximum intensity projection peripheral CT angiography image of artery calcification. Notable vertical symmetry in the calcification is observed. Both superficial femoral arteries are occluded, with a femoral to popliteal bypass on the left leg (*white arrow*). **b** Axial CT images through the mid-superficial femoral artery. Asymmetrical distribution of plaque calcification (*red arrow*). **c** Histological section of a coronary artery with a thrombus overlying an intact eccentric plaque. Area of disease-free wall (*red arrow*). Panel **c** reproduced from [12]

any atherosclerotic changes. A second important finding can be made from angio CT images—namely, disease is not uniformly distributed along a defined arterial segment; rather, we see mostly spotty or patchy distribution of calcification (Fig. 1.1). In addition, we find no calcification in any of the visceral arteries, nor in the deep femoral artery beyond 1–2 cm from their offspring from the common femoral artery. Thus, we see symmetries between left and right iliac and femoral arteries, asymmetry in the circumferential distribution, and negligible symmetry of the atherosclerotic process for defined segments of the arterial tree of the lower extremity. Comparing the extent of atherosclerosis within the entire arterial tree, the lower extremity commonly exhibits a significantly higher burden of the disease than the upper extremity. Also well known, there is segmental preference, with larger arteries systematically showing much more disease compared to small vessels, including a **continuous decline in calcification with decreasing diameter**.

These observations, however, came secondary to surgical observations during both coronary bypass surgery and surgical revascularization in peripheral vascular disease. The findings were similar—both calcific stenosis of the carotid artery or femoral artery bifurcation are almost never unilateral and there is usually no atherosclerosis in the deep femoral artery. Second, during coronary bypass surgery, the circumferential expression of atherosclerosis may be extremely variable, with the incised artery often showing a very thin-walled anterior surface together with a prominent thick-walled posterior wall. Third, and also known to every cardiac surgeon the world over, **the mammary artery, with very few exceptions, is always free from atherosclerosis.** So too are intramural stretches of coronary arteries, which always remain free from disease even in patients with extreme calcification and noncalcified lesions in the coronary segments proximal and distal to its intramural segment. These radiological and surgical-pathologic findings are definitely not new, yet they inform fundamental aspects of the pathogenesis of atherosclerosis and argue against the dogma that atherosclerosis is a generalized disease.

Ideas surrounding the mechanisms involved in atherosclerosis development have gone through some noteworthy phases. Historical, current, sometimes reinvented, and nullified hypotheses on the pathogenesis of the disease demonstrate the scientific uncertainty of the process of atherosclerosis and its initiation. Even before the age of risk factor identification, the lipid hypothesis postulated the link between blood cholesterol levels and atherosclerotic disease. Anitschow's cholesterol feeding experiments in rabbits [13] were the first to implicate dietary fats in the disease process—an idea that was later picked up on in the 1950s, but has come under recent scrutiny [14, 15]. In the age before antibiotics, the infectious theory of atherosclerosis was another favored hypothesis [16–20] which resurfaced in the 1980s [21], but which faded from popularity upon failed antibiotic drug trials to treat atherosclerosis. In the late nineteenth century, the Heidelberg school of pathologists worked diligently on vascular and blood flow mechanics with regard to their influence on arterial wall thickening [22]. The sheer stress theory of atherosclerosis has undergone a metamorphosis from "too high is bad" (1980s-the end of the 1990s) [23–25] to "too low is bad" (2000-now) [26–28]. And lastly, the inflammatory nature of atherosclerotic plaques was recognized in the mid-nineteenth century by Rudolf Virchow who noted, "In some, particularly violent cases the softening manifests itself even in the arteries not as the consequence of a really fatty process, but as a direct product of inflammation" [29]. The inflammatory hypothesis of atherosclerosis fell by the wayside during the heady days of the diet–heart hypothesis but has had a recent resurgence as a preeminent mechanism of disease progression.

When thinking of atherosclerosis, we think it's important to dispel two important misconceptions. First, **atherosclerosis is not restricted to humans**, as it is prevalent in a wide array of animals—herbivores, omnivores, and carnivores alike [30, 31]. How then do risk factors like obesity, physical inactivity, and a diet high in saturated fats make sense in this context? Secondly, contrary to popular belief, atherosclerosis is actually an ancient disease as it has been found to be prevalent in many mummies [32–34]. Most notably, the HORUS Study found evidence of atherosclerosis in mummies from Egyptian, Peruvian, Ancestral Puebloan, and Unangan populations, representing individuals from multiple time periods, disparate geographical regions, with different diets. The disease was observed in 37% of all mummies, whose average age was 37. The finding of atherosclerosis in animals and ancient mummies counters the notion that atherosclerosis is a disease necessarily associated with a modern lifestyle, a particular diet, or simply living into old age.

Most textbooks and other comprehensive sources of medical knowledge file well-known risk factors under the chapter "atherosclerosis pathogenesis", rather than describing the pathophysiology of disease development. But while hypothesis-generating, what do risk factors really tell us about how the disease is initiated? All researchers had convincing evidence in their eyes from either clinical observation or experimental data to convey their hypothesis to the medical community. Yet, none of them tried to correlate their concept with the convincing data on the local and regional expression of the disease in humans. In general, all of the systemic risk factors should affect all arterial blood vessels in the same way—upper extremity, lower extremity, small arteries, large arteries, branched vessels, and conducting arteries, mammary arteries and left anterior descending coronary arteries, young arteries and old. But they do not. Against this background of identical systemic risk factors for the disease in affected and non-diseased arterial segments, **there are defined anatomic locations within the arterial tree with advanced and dangerous lesions** (in the clinical jargon "widow makers"), with other segments always remaining free from disease. This recurring clinicopathological presentation of the disease raises questions of significant critical interest regarding the pathogenesis of atherosclerosis, namely,

What are the local factors that protect certain areas of the arterial tree from atherosclerosis in the face of the systemic effects of detrimental factors?

What are the local factors that render other areas of the arterial tree more vulnerable (susceptible) to atherosclerosis?

This book proposes a single unifying mechanism of disease development that would account for these observations, as well as explain why the well-known risk factors actually put individuals at higher risk. This pathomechanism holds true not only for obstructive atheroma formation but also for aneurysmal dilatation as well as for aortic and peripheral artery dissection. When seen through this lens, new preventive and therapeutic opportunities can be envisioned.

References

1. Defense USD. DoD News Briefing–Secretary Rumsfeld and Gen. Myers. 2002. http://archive.defense.gov/Transcripts/Transcript.aspx?TranscriptID=2636. Accessed 20 Sept 2018.
2. Marchand F. Über Arteriosklerose. Verhandlungen des Kongresses für Inn Medizin 21 Kongress Leipzig; 1904. p. 23–59.
3. WHO. Projections of mortality and causes of death, 2015 and 2030. 2012. http://www.who.int/healthinfo/global_burden_disease/projections/en/.
4. Ophüls W. Arteriosclerosis cardiovascular disease: their relation to infectious diseases. 1st ed. California: Standford University Press; 1921.
5. Winternitz MC, Thomas RMM, LeCompte P. The biology of arteriosclerosis. Springfield, IL: Charles C Thomas; 1938.
6. Creech O. A surgeon's view of atherosclerosis. Am Heart J. 1957;54:641–2.
7. French JE. Atherosclerosis in relation to the structure and function of the arterial intima, with special reference to th endothelium. Int Rev Exp Pathol. 1966;5:253–353.
8. Hauss WH, Bauch HJ, Schulte H. Adrenaline and noradrenaline as possible chemical mediators in the pathogenesis of arteriosclerosis. Ann NY Acad Sci. 1990;598:91–101.
9. Nakashima Y, Wight TN, Sueishi K. Early atherosclerosis in humans: role of diffuse intimal thickening and extracellular matrix proteoglycans. Cardiovasc Res. 2008;79:14–23. https://doi.org/10.1093/cvr/cvn099.
10. National Heart, Lung and BI Atherosclerosis. https://www.nhlbi.nih.gov/health/health-topics/topics/atherosclerosis/causes. Accessed 18 Sept 2018.
11. Hansen T, Wikström J, Johansson LO, et al. The prevalence and quantification of atherosclerosis in an elderly population assessed by whole-body magnetic resonance angiography. Arterioscler Thromb Vasc Biol. 2007;27:649–54. https://doi.org/10.1161/01.ATV.0000255310.47940.3b.
12. Burke AP, Farb A, Malcom GT, et al. Effect of risk factors on the mechanism of acute thrombosis and sudden coronary death in women. Circulation. 1998;97:2110–6.
13. Anitschow NN, Chalatow S. Ueber den Gehalt normaler und atheromatoser Aorten an Cholesterol und Cholesterinester. Zentrbl Allg Pathol Pathol Anat. 1913;24:1–9.
14. Stehbens WE. Coronary heart disease, hypercholesterolemia, and atherosclerosis I. False premises. Exp Mol Pathol. 2001;70:103–19. https://doi.org/10.1006/exmp.2000.2340.
15. Stehbens WE. Coronary heart disease, hypercholesterolemia, and atherosclerosis II. Misrepresented data. Exp Mol Pathol. 2001;70:120–39. https://doi.org/10.1006/exmp.2000.2339.
16. Thayer W, Brush C. The relation of acute infections and arteriosclerosis. JAMA. 1904;43:583–4.
17. Thayer W. On the late effects of typhoid fever on the heart and vessels. Am J Med Sci. 1904;77:391–422.
18. Gilbert L. Artérites infectieuses expérimentales. Compt rend Soc biol. 1889.
19. Crocq. Contribution a L'étude expérimentale des artérites infectieuses. Arch méd Exp. 1894;6:583.

20. Klotz. The experimental production of arteriosclerosis. Br Med J. 1906;2:1767.
21. Fabricant CG, Fabricant J, Litrenta MM, Minick CR. Virus-induced atherosclerosis. J Exp Med. 1978;148:335–40.
22. Thoma R. Über die Abhängigkeit der Bindegewebsneubildung in der Arterienintima von den mechanischen Bedingungen des Blutumlaufs. Virchows Arch. 1883;93:443–505.
23. Diamond SL, Eskin SG, McIntire LV. Fluid flow stimulates tissue plasminogen activator secretion by cultured human endothelial cells. Science. 1989;243:1483–5.
24. Kosaki K, Ando J, Korenaga R, et al. Fluid shear stress increases the production of granulocyte-macrophage colony-stimulating factor by endothelial cells via mRNA stabilization. Circ Res. 1998;82:794–802.
25. Thubrikar MJ, Robicsek F. Pressure-induced arterial wall stress and atherosclerosis. Ann Thorac Surg. 1995;59:1594–603.
26. Shaaban AM, Duerinckx AJ. Wall shear stress and early atherosclerosis: a review. AJR Am J Roentgenol. 2000;174:1657–65. https://doi.org/10.2214/ajr.174.6.1741657.
27. Cunningham KS, Gotlieb AI. The role of shear stress in the pathogenesis of atherosclerosis. Lab Invest. 2005;85:9–23. https://doi.org/10.1038/labinvest.3700215.
28. Stone PH, Maehara A, Coskun AU, et al. Role of low endothelial shear stress and plaque characteristics in the prediction of nonculprit major adverse cardiac events: the PROSPECT study. JACC Cardiovasc Imaging. 2018;11:462–71. https://doi.org/10.1016/j.jcmg.2017.01.031.
29. Virchow R. Cellular pathology. 1860.
30. Adams CW. Arteriosclerosis in man, other mammals and birds. Biol Rev Camb Philos Soc. 1964;39:372–423.
31. Dahme EG. Atherosclerosis and arteriosclerosis in domestic animals. Ann NY Acad Sci. 1965;127:657–70. https://doi.org/10.1164/arrd.1978.118.6.1101.
32. Sandison AT. Degenerative vascular disease in the Egyptian mummy. Med Hist. 1962;6:77–81.
33. Thompson RC, Allam AH, Lombardi GP, et al. Atherosclerosis across 4000 years of human history: the Horus study of four ancient populations. Lancet (London, England). 2013;381:1211–22. https://doi.org/10.1016/S0140-6736(13)60598-X.
34. Allam AH, Thompson RC, Wann LS, et al. Atherosclerosis in ancient Egyptian mummies: the Horus study. JACC Cardiovasc Imaging. 2011;4:315–27. https://doi.org/10.1016/j.jcmg.2011.02.002.

Chapter 2
Atherosclerosis Risk Factors

2.1 A Short History of the Term "Risk Factor"

Cardiovascular epidemiology began in earnest in the 1930s with Anitschow presenting at the International Society of Geographical Pathology on the frequency of atherosclerotic lesions across countries and by social class and occupation [1]. In 1947, Ancel Keys initiated his now famous prospective study on coronary heart disease in Minnesota businessmen [2]. Around the same time, the seminal Framingham Heart Study began. Its objective was to discover the common factors or characteristics that contribute to cardiovascular disease by monitoring disease development in a large group of participants over a long time period [3–6]. The now widely used term "risk factor" originated from this study and was defined as a variable that is causally associated with an increased rate of the disease and that is an independent and significant predictor of the risk of developing the disease [7]. After a 4-year follow-up, the Framingham Heart Study reported age- and sex-related differences in coronary heart disease and identified the first three major risk factors: hypertension, hypercholesteremia, and obesity [5]. Since then, this study and others have gone on to identify what are considered today to be well-established or "classical" risk factors for atherosclerosis including inherent risk factors that result from unavoidable genetic or physical conditions, comorbidities, as well as modifiable lifestyle factors (Fig. 2.1). These studies were then the impetus for large public health initiatives against smoking in the 1960s, hypertension in the 1970s, and hypercholesterolemia in the 1980s. When speaking about risk factors, however, it is important to keep in mind that their identification reveals little about their causal connection, if any, to disease.

© Springer Nature Switzerland AG 2019
A. Haverich and E. C. Boyle, *Atherosclerosis Pathogenesis and Microvascular Dysfunction*, https://doi.org/10.1007/978-3-030-20245-3_2

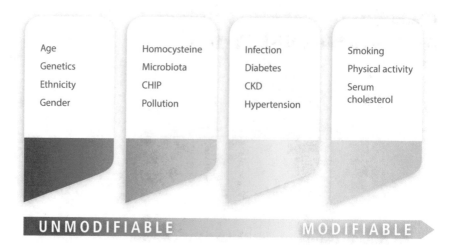

Fig. 2.1 Classification of atherosclerosis risk factors ranging from unmodifiable to modifiable. CHIP, clonal hematopoiesis of indeterminate potential; CKD, chronic kidney disease

2.2   Classical Risk Factors

Some of the classical risk factors associated with atherosclerosis are inherent and unmodifiable such as gender, ethnicity, and family history. For example, it's known that men are more likely to develop and die of heart disease than women; however, this changes when women reach menopause [8]. African Americans and Asians have a higher risk of coronary disease than Caucasians [9]. There is also an important genetic component to atherosclerosis, as family history also affects susceptibility to disease [10, 11]. For instance, if a first-degree male relative is diagnosed with heart disease before the age of 55, or a first-degree female family member before the age of 65, an individual has a 2.5–7 times higher risk of developing heart disease [12]. Children of parents who have had premature myocardial infarction have abnormal arteries and demonstrate the first signs of atherosclerosis development at an early age compared to subjects without a family history of chronic heart disease [11, 13].

Several concomitant diseases, otherwise known as comorbidities, also influence the risk of developing atherosclerosis. A number of large epidemiological studies have identified an important connection between cardiovascular disease and diabetes, with a higher risk association in women than in men [14–19]. The prevalence of diabetes worldwide was estimated to be 6.4% of the population in 2010 [20]. Diabetics have a 2–8 times higher risk of coronary heart disease than healthy individuals [21], which is related to glycemic regulation and glucose intolerance [22, 23]. Moreover, other risk factors for cardiovascular disease such as hypertension, high blood cholesterol, and obesity occur more often in diabetic individuals.

Chronic kidney disease (CKD) is another risk factor for heart disease [24–26]. In fact, CKD patients are more likely to die of cardiovascular disease than to develop kidney failure [25, 27]. Dialysis patients die of cardiovascular disease 10–20 times more often than the general population [24]. The Framingham Heart Study was among the first to assess mild renal insufficiency and its association with death and adverse cardiovascular events in the general population [28]. An independent, graded association was found between low estimated glomerular flow rate and the risk of cardiovascular events in a large, low-risk, community-based population [29]. Kidney disease is invariably associated with inflammation and hypertension, and is frequently associated with dyslipidemia, which in turn accelerate the progression of atherosclerosis.

The Framingham Heart study was the first to identify obesity as a significant independent predictor of heart disease [30] while more recent studies show that, in particular, it is associated with a higher risk of atherosclerosis [31]. Importantly, obesity is a major upstream driver of other established risk factors for atherosclerosis such as hypertension, dyslipidemia, and diabetes. However, even metabolically healthy obese individuals are at higher risk of developing coronary heart disease, cerebrovascular disease, and heart failure than normal weight metabolically healthy individuals [32]. Weight distribution also influences disease risk in that even normal weight individuals who have substantial intra-abdominal fat ("big belly") are at a greater risk of coronary artery disease [33]. Studies in twins have shown there is a genetic component to obesity with hereditability estimated to be 40–70% [34], with more than 20 obesity susceptibility loci identified. Physical activity is one of the primary ways to counteract obesity, and there is significant evidence that lack of physical activity also puts individuals at a higher risk of cardiovascular disease [35–38]. While obesity and lack of physical activity are strongly correlated, even physically active overweight or obese people can significantly reduce their risk of disease with regular physical activity [39, 40].

The Framingham Heart Study defined hypertension as a blood pressure of $\geq 160/95$ mmHg. It found that the incidence of coronary heart disease was 4 times higher among patients with high blood pressure than in normotensive individuals [5] with the systolic value playing a more important role than diastolic pressure [41]. Since then, elevated blood pressure has been consistently associated with a higher risk of atherosclerosis and cardiovascular disease in prospective population studies [42–45]. Moreover, in randomized trials, treatment of high blood pressure with antihypertensive drugs lowers the risk of cardiovascular disease [46–49]. Today, the American Heart Association estimates that 34% of American adults have hypertension [20]. Seventy-six percent of these patients use antihypertensive drugs, but only about half of them have their blood pressure under control. It is estimated that 70% of men and 50% of women who have high blood pressure at middle age will develop cardiovascular events by the age of 85 [50]. Even high-normal blood pressure ($\geq 130–139/85–89$ mmHg) doubles the risk of heart disease [51]. Hypertension is an important risk factor that has inherent as well as modifiable aspects. Genetics as well as certain comorbidities put individuals at higher risk of having high blood pressure. On the other hand, modifiable lifestyle aspects such as stress, obesity, lack of physical activity, and smoking also increase hypertension.

No other personal choice has a more negative impact on cardiovascular health than smoking. Adults who smoke die on average 13–14 years earlier than non-smokers, with nearly half of the premature mortality associated with cardiovascular disease. It has been known since the 1940/50s that cigarette smoking is associated with heart disease [52–55]. Persons who smoke more than 20 cigarettes a day are 3 times as likely to develop heart disease [56]. Not only is active smoking dangerous, but so too is secondhand exposure [57–59]. Intimal thickening, which some consider to be an early phase of atherosclerosis, is significantly associated with smoking [60]. Some of the negative effects of smoking are reversible as individuals who stop smoking after infarction decrease their risk of having another coronary event [61].

2.3 Controversial Risk Factors

2.3.1 Dietary Cholesterol

The Russian immunologist and 1908 Nobel Prize winner Élie Metchnikoff proposed that an excess of protein in the diet was potentially toxic and accelerated the aging process. Inspired by the hypothesis of Metchnikoff, a young experimental pathologist working at the Military Medical Academy in St. Petersburg, Alexander Ignatowski, carried out experiments on rabbits, feeding them large amounts of meat, eggs, and milk. He found that rabbits fed this high protein diet had, in addition to changes in the liver, spleen, and kidneys, striking arterial lesions which resembled human atherosclerosis. Later, he progressively narrowed things down and showed that simply feeding cholesterol purified from egg yolks induced vascular damage. Following this work, his colleague Nikolai Anitschow tested the idea that cholesterol in particular was responsible, and began experiments feeding rabbits purified cholesterol. He found that cholesterol feeding induced lesions in the arteries that looked similar to atherosclerosis in human autopsy specimens. Accordingly, he firmly believed that dietary cholesterol was the cause of atherosclerosis. He revised his theory slightly in 1924, and consequently, the "cholesterol hypothesis" or "lipid hypothesis" was conceived—the concept that high cholesterol levels in the blood were necessary for deposition of lipids in the blood vessel wall [62]. **Anitschow's work met criticism concerning the rabbits' extremely high serum cholesterol values (between 500 and 1000 mg/dL).** In addition, comparable results were never achieved in non-herbivores such as the dog or rat.

Although he worked in renowned laboratories in Germany and Austria where he met scientists from all over the world, Anitschow's work remained largely unknown for many years. The only publication in English before 1950 was a chapter in the first edition of Cowdry's *Arteriosclerosis* (1933). Not until 1950, did Anitschow's work on cholesterol and atherosclerosis gain worldwide recognition due to a publication by John Gofman called, "The role of lipids and lipoproteins in atherosclerosis" [63, 64]. In it, Gofman specifically states that Anitschow was the first to discover the association between dietary cholesterol and vascular disease and using Anitschow's methods, his group confirmed and extended his findings. Gofman's group was the first to successfully use analytic ultracentrifugation to fractionate serum into a low-density lipoprotein (LDL) and a high-density lipoprotein (HDL) cholesterol fraction [65]. Using this technique, they showed that the low-density portion was highly correlated to atherosclerosis in both rabbits and humans [63, 66, 67]. This kindled immense interest in cholesterol-induced atherosclerosis research and in Anitschow's work, 40 years after the Russian pathologist's first discoveries on this disease.

The implication that high serum cholesterol resulted from dietary intake of cholesterol was quickly assumed. In 1952, Kinsell et al. showed that replacing animal fats with vegetable fats lowered serum cholesterol levels in human subjects [68]. In 1954, Ahrens et al. demonstrated that this was because vegetable fats are unsaturated [69]. Around the same time, a nutritional scientist from the University of Minnesota named Ancel Keys, was on sabbatical leave at Oxford University when he traveled to Italy [70]. A colleague there claimed that workers in Naples seldom had heart attacks. Upon further investigation, he saw that they rarely ate meat and butter, while in more affluent people, where heart attacks were sometimes seen, meat and butter were prevalent. This triggered his interest in the "dietary hypothesis" of coronary heart disease. In 1953, Keys presented the relationship between mortality from degenerative heart disease and fat calories as a percentage of total calories in the diet of populations from six different countries (Japan, Italy, England and Wales, Australia, Canada, and USA) [71]. For men aged 55–59, a strong relationship between fat calories as a percentage of dietary intake and deaths from heart disease was apparent. Therefore, Keys' conclusion was that diet was the primary factor contributing to blood lipids [72]. Keys' conclusion, however, came under immediate harsh criticism from Yerushalmy and Hilleboe, who unlike Keys, presented data available from 22 different countries [73]. In their paper, they set out "to investigate the association between dietary fat and heart disease mortality in all countries for which information is available," and concluded, "It is immediately obvious that the inclusion of all the countries greatly reduces the apparent association."

Undeterred, Keys launched the Seven Countries Study in 1958. It was a massive clinical trial that prospectively examined the connection between lifestyle, diet, and the prevalence of cardiovascular disease in middle-aged men from the United States, Japan, Greece, Yugoslavia, Italy, Finland, and the Netherlands [70, 74–77]. These countries were presumed to have been chosen due to their different lifestyles, eating habits, risk factor levels, as well as incidence of and mortality from chronic heart disease. Others have suggested the choice was partly made on the basis of convenience and previous collaborations [73, 78, 79]. **Keys and the Seven Countries Study have come under intense criticism due to their**

inability to justify the choice of these seven countries and how they may have been "cherry-picked" based on previous results [80]. However, even if all countries are included, there is still an association between fat intake and heart disease, even if it is not quite as pronounced [81].

The **Framingham Study** that had been initiated by the NIH at the same time as the Seven Countries Study also found a correlation between serum cholesterol and cardiovascular disease [5, 6]. However, they found **no link between diet and serum cholesterol levels**. A 30-year follow-up identified an association only between blood cholesterol and overall mortality or death from cardiovascular disease in individuals under age 50 [82]. **In older individuals, falling serum cholesterol levels actually correlated with an overall *increase* in the cardiovascular disease death rate. In fact, for each 1 mg/dL per year drop in serum cholesterol, there was an 11% increase in both the overall death rate and death due to cardiovascular illness**.

The Minnesota Coronary Experiment was the largest randomized, controlled dietary trial investigating cholesterol lowering by the replacement of saturated fat with vegetable oils [83]. Nine thousand individuals from a mental hospital and a nursing home were studied between 1968 and 1973. Frantz et al. found a reduction in serum cholesterol concentrations in the group substituting saturated fats with vegetable oils but no significant difference in cardiovascular events, cardiovascular death, or overall mortality. However, the authors concluded a positive trend that they postulated could become significant in a larger study. Despite the fact that the trial's results were not significant, Frantz was convinced that reducing saturated fats was crucial to prevent heart disease [84].

Over the years, more and more studies have connected dietary cholesterol to atherosclerosis [85–87], yet several cardiologists and nutritionists remained skeptical as they felt it had not been proven [88–90]. William Stehbens argued that the cholesterol–heart disease hypothesis was based on false premises such as the misuse of coronary heart disease as an equivalent to coronary atherosclerosis, false mortality rates, biased age selection, and "overzealous investigators" [91–93]. The medical community was divided [94]. A large, randomized, double-blind study on the effect of lowering plasma cholesterol with medication was initiated. The NIH sponsored "Coronary Primary Prevention Trial" showed a statistically significant decrease in cardiovascular endpoints after lowering blood cholesterol with medication. All study participants (±cholesterol-lowering medication) were put on a cholesterol-restricted diet, and therefore, the study did not directly address the impact of dietary-induced cholesterol lowering. Despite this, following the publication of the study, a consensus conference was convened by the NIH that recommended dietary cholesterol reduction and eating a low-fat diet favoring unsaturated fats [94, 95]. The idea that cholesterol caused atherosclerosis became mainstream in the 1990s. **However, cholesterol does not predict the degree of atherosclerosis at autopsy [96, 97] and does not correlate with the degree of coronary calcification [98] or coronary or peripheral atherosclerosis [99–101]**.

More recently, Ramdsen et al. reexamined studies on serum cholesterol-reducing diets where saturated fats were replaced by linoleic acid [102]. This included a reevaluation of the raw data from the Minnesota Coronary Experiment that were never fully published. Similar to Frantz et al. [83], they found replacing saturated fats led to lower serum cholesterol levels, but did not improve mortality, and there was no benefit for preventing coronary atherosclerosis. Interestingly, Ramdsen et al. discovered a 22% *higher* mortality risk associated with each 30 mg/dL reduction of serum cholesterol. This was also confirmed in an evaluation of 19 cohort studies in the elderly. **Higher LDL levels *inversely* correlated with mortality in people over the age of 60, a finding that is inconsistent with the cholesterol hypothesis** [103].

The cholesterol hypothesis proposes that high concentrations of LDL cholesterol in the blood cause atherosclerosis, and if correct, one would predict that lowering LDL cholesterol should reverse or at least stop atherosclerosis. Active cholesterol-lowering therapy for atherosclerosis became a standard medical practice after studies with cholesterol biosynthesis inhibiting drugs (statins) showed a reduction in deaths due to coronary heart disease [104]. Ross et al. demonstrated a 20–30% decline in major coronary events and death in patients treated with statins [105]. Using statins in secondary prevention seems to be even more effective than in primary prevention [106]. It was suggested that the initially recommended LDL level of less than 100 mg/dL be reduced to less than 70 mg/dL [107–109]. A study employing 80 mg atorvastatin to reduce concentrations to this low level demonstrated a benefit in total major cardiovascular events in patients with stable coronary disease. However, death from any cause did not differ, and intensive lipid-lowering therapy was associated with a higher incidence of elevated alanine aminotransferase and/or aspartate levels. And in high-risk primary prevention, statins did not reduce all-cause mortality [110].

DuBroff criticized studies with statins as being falsely interpreted, because although the mortality due to coronary heart disease was reduced by the drug, the overall mortality often was not [110, 111]. The decline in cardiovascular deaths in countries like the US where the use of statins is high is considered by some to be proof that statins are effective. However, other risk factors, such as smoking, which have also declined, could have a concomitant effect. Adopting a Mediterranean diet was equally or more successful than lipid-lowering drugs in several studies [112–114], raising the question: what are the true benefits of statins?

New serum cholesterol-lowering drugs target a protein in the liver called proprotein convertase subtilisin kexin 9 (PCSK9). PCSK9 binds to the LDL receptor (LDLR) and results in its intracellular degradation. If PCSK9 is inhibited, more LDLRs are recycled back onto the cell surface and are therefore available to remove more LDL particles from the blood. Blocking PCSK9 with antibodies [115–117] or inhibiting protein synthesis with small interfering RNA (siRNA) nanoparticles [118] has been shown to reduce serum LDL by 40–60% compared to controls. A single dose of 300 mg of siRNA nanoparticles was effective in lowering LDL for 6 months with no serious adverse events [119]. In both therapeutic approaches, the majority of patients were also taking statins, which indicates that there may be an overall synergistic effect on lowering LDL cholesterol levels [120].

2.3.2 Infection

"The sclerosis of old age may simply be a summation of lesions arising from infectious or metabolic toxins." (Frothingham 1911) [121]

"There is every indication that the production of tissue in the intima is the result of a direct irritation of that tissue by the presence of infection or toxins." (Klotz and Manning 1911) [122]

Infection is one of the oldest etiological hypotheses of atherosclerosis. Interestingly, Anitschow, while defending his cholesterol theory during a fellowship stay with Aschoff in Heidelberg, encouraged his colleagues in St. Petersburg to continue their studies on the infectious origin of arteriosclerosis [64]. Clinical observers at the end of the nineteenth and the beginning of the twentieth century such as Martin (1881), Thérèse (1893), Simnitzky (1903), Wiesel (1906), and Zinserling (1913) studied arterial autopsy specimens of children and young adults who had died of various infectious diseases [123–127]. They observed pathological changes of the media in the aorta and smaller arteries and concluded pathogenic microorganisms were responsible. In 1891, Huchard considered that the acute infectious diseases of childhood were largely responsible for the arteriosclerosis of adult life. In 1904, Thayer found a high frequency of arterial lesions in patients who died from typhoid fever and a high prevalence of arteriosclerotic radial arteries in those who survived [128, 129]. **Sir William Osler was also a believer of the infectious cause of arteriosclerosis stating in his book, "Modern Medicine", that in scarlet fever, measles, diphtheria, smallpox, and influenza cases, arterial degeneration occurs with great frequency** [130]. The Danish pathologist Faber published a whole volume on arteriosclerosis in 1908, where he indicated a locoregional affection of arteries according to the site of infection [131]. In addition to human autopsy material, he included animal studies where he observed increased rates of abdominal aortic arteriosclerosis in 2-year-old calves with udder tuberculosis compared to those free of this infection. Meanwhile, William Ophüls, pathologist and the first Dean of the Stanford University Medical School, found the association between infection and arteriosclerosis so compelling that he wrote an in-depth review on the topic in 1921 [132].

Meanwhile, corroborative observations in animal models began to accumulate. As early as 1889, fatty sclerotic changes in the aorta of rabbits were observed after injection with pathogenic bacteria either alone or in combination with slight mechanical injury to the arterial wall [133–136]. These initial animal experiments, resulting in reproducible initiation of the arteriosclerotic process in various European (France, Italy, Switzerland, and Germany) laboratories, clearly demonstrated the ability of certain bacteria to induce the disease process.

Early epidemiological studies found that acute cardiovascular events peaked during flu and pneumonia epidemics suggesting the importance of infection in heart disease [137, 138]. However, infection as a pathogenic factor for atherosclerosis waned from popularity when studies like the Seven Countries Study and the Framingham Study led to a shift to cholesterol-based research. Interest in an infectious basis for atherosclerosis was rekindled when Fabricant demonstrated that a chicken herpes virus could induce atherosclerotic changes in chickens [139]. Since then, other infectious agents, including respiratory pathogens (*Chlamydia pneumoniae* and influenza virus), periodontal pathogens (*Porphyromonas gingivalis, Aggregatibacter actinomycetemcomitans*), a gastric pathogen (*Helicobacter pylori*), and cytomegalovirus have been reported to accelerate atherosclerotic lesion progression in animal models of atherosclerosis [140–157].

Simultaneously, numerous (sero)epidemiological studies accumulated that supported a role for infection in cardiovascular disease [158]. Antibody titers to specific pathogens were found to correlate with atherosclerosis risk [148, 149, 159–166], cardiovascular disease [161, 167], and cardiovascular disease mortality [168]. However, there were also contradictory data reporting no relationship between seropositivity and cardiovascular disease [169–172]. One of the strongest links between acute infection and cardiovascular events is the link between myocardial infarction and respiratory infections, especially influenza and community-acquired pneumonia [173, 174]. There is a clear higher incidence of acute myocardial infarction in the winter, a time when respiratory infections are common [175, 176]. A meta-analysis of 16 epidemiological studies showed a significant association between recent respiratory infection and cardiac arrest [177]. **The fact that influenza and pneumococcal vaccination significantly reduces heart disease is another sign that acute infection is involved** [178–181].

Some of the strongest associations between chronic infection and cardiovascular disease involve *C. pneumoniae* and *H. pylori* [182–187]. There is also strong evidence that periodontal disease, a chronic multibacterial infection of the gums, is associated with cardiovascular disease [149, 188, 189]. Poor dental health is related to acute myocardial infarction and the risk of coronary heart disease increases along with the severity of periodontitis [188, 190–193]. A Danish study found that patients with periodontitis had a risk of cardiovascular disease that was twice as high as patients with healthy gums [194]. Recently, a Dutch cross-sectional analysis of 60,174 participants concluded that periodontitis is an independent risk factor for atherosclerosis [195]. Individuals with periodontal disease have increased systemic inflammation, endothelial dysfunction, and carotid intima–media thickness. Treatment of periodontal disease alone has been shown to significantly reduce these surrogate markers of atherosclerotic plaque development [196–198]. Even in the much milder case of experimentally induced gingivitis in young healthy patients, dental hygiene can almost completely reverse the increased systemic markers of inflammation [199].

Altogether, research demonstrates that atherosclerosis is associated with a number of different pathogens. This brings us to an important debate surrounding the infectious origin of atherosclerosis which is: do pathogens directly cause atherosclerosis or is it an indirect effect caused by the systemic inflammation they induce? In support of pathogens directly inducing atherosclerosis, numerous pathogens have been detected within atherosclerotic plaques including

C. pneumoniae, H. pylori, Mycoplasma pneumoniae, Enterobacter hormaechei, cytomegalovirus, hepatitis C virus, human immunodeficiency virus, herpes simplex viruses, Epstein–Barr virus, and enteroviruses (Fig. 2.2) [149, 200–211]. Consistent with an individual's seropositivity, corresponding pathogens including periodontal pathogens such as *A. actinomycetemcomitans, Bacteroides forsythus,* and *P. gingivalis* have also been isolated from atherosclerotic plaques [212–216]. With the advent of deep sequencing technology, more and more microbes are being found within diseased arteries [217–224]. With the multitude of microorganisms being located in atherosclerotic plaques, the idea of one's lifetime "**infectious burden**" was suggested to be responsible for the disease. Over time, it appears that the number of infections not only correlated with atherosclerosis but also with disease severity [162, 225–227]. Elkind et al. (Northern

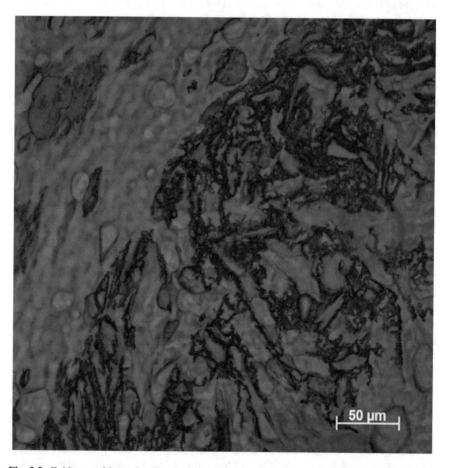

Fig. 2.2 Evidence of bacteria directly in human atherosclerotic plaques. Fluorescence in situ hybridization of an atherosclerotic plaque sample using an *H. pylori*-specific probe (purple). Reproduced from [223]

Manhattan Study) reported an association between infectious burden and maximum carotid plaques thickness [228]. Therefore, could the association between atherosclerosis and one or multiple infections be an indirect effect of generalized inflammation caused by these infections? Certainly, it was an idea that has been proposed before, but it wasn't until more recently that the "inflammation hypothesis" of atherosclerosis came once again to the forefront (see Inflammation: Just Another Risk Factor or a Unifying Concept?).

If pathogens are associated with cardiovascular disease, eradicating these pathogens should stop or at least improve atherosclerosis progression. Several studies investigating the antibiotic treatment of *C. pneumoniae* and *H. pylori* infections for secondary prevention of atherosclerosis have shown a positive effect on several cardiovascular disease markers [229–235]. For example, depletion of *H. pylori* led to a decrease in oxidative stress, myeloperoxidase activity, and fat mass—all biomarkers of atherosclerosis [234]. In several other small-scale trials utilizing non-invasive measurements of aortic aneurysm growth and carotid artery wall thickness, antibiotics showed a positive effect on peripheral vascular disease symptoms and restenosis after stent placement in coronary arteries. While these smaller studies showed a benefit of antibiotic therapy, large clinical trials like WIZARD [236], ACES [237], CLARICOR [238], and a large meta-analysis evaluating 13 trials with 12,491 treated patients [239] failed to show any long-term benefit of antibiotic treatment on cardiovascular diseases. While many people following these clinical intervention trials quickly closed the book on the hope that antibiotics could be used in secondary prevention of cardiovascular disease [239], these trials also drew harsh criticism [229, 240, 241]. Chronic *C. pneumoniae* and *H. pylori* infections are notoriously difficult to treat with antibiotics. For example, *Chlamydia* has both an intracellular persistent phase and an extracellular non-replicating form that are not susceptible to antibiotics. Current therapy for eradication of *H. pylori* consists of a proton pump inhibitor to prevent antibiotic degradation in the acidic stomach environment in combination with two to four different antibiotics given sequentially or simultaneously [242, 243]. Despite this, the efficacy of *H. pylori* treatment is often inadequately low [244]. **The limited courses of antibiotics given in the cardiovascular disease clinical trials were said to be entirely unsuitable to treat these chronic infections.** Another suggested explanation for why the clinical trials failed was that antibiotics were given at a late stage in the atherosclerotic disease process, perhaps too late to significantly alter disease outcomes. Given the aforementioned positive effects of influenza vaccination on cardiovascular disease, the future development of both *C. pneumoniae* and *H. pylori* vaccines will be of great interest for their ability to prevent cardiovascular disease.

2.3.3 Homocysteine

Homocysteine is a natural by-product of methionine degradation [245, 246]. The normal range of total homocysteine in the blood ranges from 5 to 15 μmol/L.

Homocysteine was first linked to atherosclerosis in 1969 when it was observed that atherosclerotic plaques are prevalent in patients with homocystinuria, an inherited disease affecting amino acid metabolism [247, 248]. Aside from being inherited, high levels of homocysteine in the blood can be acquired. Smoking, folic acid or vitamin B deficiency, as well as drinking coffee can cause higher levels of plasma homocysteine. A large number of epidemiological studies have confirmed the association between high plasma concentrations of homocysteine and the prevalence of cardiovascular events [249]. Still, there is an ongoing debate as to whether homocysteine should be viewed as a risk factor or simply a biomarker since several randomized controlled trials and meta-analyses have shown that homocysteine-lowering interventions do not reduce the occurrence of cardiovascular events [250–255]. However, the majority of these interventional trials were conducted in patients with preexisting cardiovascular disease. To solidify homocysteine as a bona fide risk factor, a large randomized controlled trial performed in low to intermediate risk patients with no previous cardiovascular disease is needed.

2.4   Emerging Risk Factors

2.4.1   Particulate Air Pollution

Air pollution is a complex mixture of gaseous, volatile, and semi-volatile substances as well as particulate matter (PM) [256]. While gaseous air pollutants can undoubtedly have serious health effects, epidemiological evidence suggests that PM has the greatest effect on human health [256–258]. Particulate matter is classified according to its average diameter: coarse particles $<10 \, \mu m$ (termed PM10), fine particles <2.5 (termed PM2.5), and ultrafine particles $<0.1 \, \mu m$ [259]. Exposure to ambient air pollution increases mortality and morbidity and shortens life expectancy [260, 261]. It is the leading cause of global disease burden and is currently the fifth-ranking mortality risk factor. Between 1990 and 2015, the Global Burden of Disease Study estimated that PM2.5 accounted for 7.6% of the global deaths and 4.2% of the global disability-adjusted life years (DALYs) [262].

A large number of epidemiological studies have shown the association between exposure to air pollution and cardiovascular disease. In the 1990s, epidemiological studies such as the Harvard Six Cities Study and American Cancer Society cohort studies drew attention to pollution as a risk factor for cardiovascular disease [259, 263, 264]. In various large epidemiological studies since, long-term exposure to PM has been linked to cardiovascular mortality [265–272], myocardial infarction [273–275], and atherosclerosis [276–289]. Even at concentrations well below the European Commission Air Quality Standard (annual mean limit of $25 \, \mu g/m^3$) exposure to PM is associated with cardiovascular disease and specific cardiovascular causes of death [268]. Meta-analyses have estimated that 7.4% of myocardial infarctions could be prevented if there was no exposure to air pollution caused by traffic [259, 290, 291]. After the ban of bituminous coal in Dublin, Ireland in the early 1990s, air quality improved almost overnight with a corresponding precipitous fall in the incidence of cardiovascular events [292]. In our own research, we've seen long-term exposure to particulate air pollution independently increases the risk of cardiac allograft vasculopathy in heart transplant patients [293]. **In addition to long-term exposure, short-term exposure to PM is associated with cardiovascular mortality** [294], myocardial infarction [295], and emergency hospitalizations [296–299]. Acute cardiovascular complications involving plaque vulnerability, thrombosis, and acute ischemic events can also be triggered by short-term exposure to particulate air pollution [300–305].

In some of these epidemiological studies, residential proximity to major roadways is used as a proxy for pollution exposure. For example, it was found that persons living near major roads have an increased risk of cardiac mortality [265, 306, 307], atherosclerosis [282, 284, 285, 308], and acute myocardial infarction [309]. In a study of 107,103 women, Hart et al. found a 6% increase in hazard ratio for sudden cardiac death for every 100 m they lived closer to a main road [306]. The accuracy of residential roadway proximity as a proxy for air pollution exposure can be debated. This estimation does not take into account temporal changes in traffic volume, the emissions of the vehicular fleet, the amount of time each participant spends at their home, or the characteristics of each home such as age, ventilation rate, and orientation relative to prevailing winds and the roadways.

Aside from epidemiologic studies, there are observations from controlled exposure experiments in animals and humans. These have the advantage that they are performed under precisely defined and reproducible conditions. The majority of these studies have been performed with inhalation of air containing combustion-derived particles (e.g., diesel exhaust particulate matter). In mice and rabbits, studies show that exposure to diesel PM influences the progression of atherosclerosis [310–314]. In humans, short-term PM exposure leads to changes in arterial hemodynamics that include acute vasoconstriction of the brachial artery [315, 316], immediate and transient increases in central arterial stiffness that increases arterial tone [317], and decreased heart rate variability [318–321]. It also results in a rise in diastolic and mean arterial pressure [322, 323], exacerbation of exercise-related myocardial infarction in men with coronary disease [324], impaired vascular vasomotor functions due to endothelial dysfunction [324, 325], and increased thrombosis by means of platelet activation and impaired fibrinolysis [326]. In a randomized, double-blind, crossover trial of domestic air purification, they found higher blood pressure, stress-related hormones, insulin resistance, and biomarkers of oxidative stress and inflammation among individuals exposed to higher levels of ambient particulate matter as well as short-term reductions in these factors following indoor air purification [327]. Thus, pollutants affect blood pressure, hormone and lipid levels, vascular function, and inflammation, similar to many other risk factors influencing cardiovascular disease. Therefore, the tremendously elevated levels of small particle air pollution seen with the rise of global urbanization is a major challenge for the future global risk of atherosclerosis.

2.4.2   Trimethylamine N-Oxide and the Intestinal Microbiota

The lumen of the human intestine hosts a vast microbial community known as the gut microbiota. With populations exceeding 100 trillion microorganisms, the gut microbiota achieves the highest cell densities recorded for any ecosystem. Commensal bacteria play crucial roles in essential vitamin production, carbohydrate degradation, signaling molecule production, and immune system function and development. Despite numerous beneficial roles in human health, there is now substantial evidence that the intestinal microbiota plays a key role in the pathophysiology of various diseases.

Stanley Hazen's group at the Cleveland Clinic was looking for proatherogenic metabolite biomarkers. In a large clinical cohort, they discovered that the presence of trimethylamine N-oxide (TMAO) in the serum could predict the risk of cardiovascular disease. Since this initial report, multiple independent cohorts have found that serum TMAO levels are linked to a higher risk of cardiovascular disease, including atherosclerosis [328–333].

Humans are not capable of producing TMAO by themselves. It turns out that the production of TMAO depends on the intestinal microbiota when they metabolize phosphatidylcholine, choline, and carnitine, most commonly found in foods like red meat, shellfish, and eggs. TMAO formation occurs via a two-step pathway [328, 331]. Following nutrient ingestion, gut microbes produce trimethylamine (TMA) which travels via the portal vein to the liver where flavin monooxygenases catalyze the conversion of TMA into TMAO. In humans, blocking TMAO synthesis by suppressing intestinal microbiota with antibiotics, leads to lower TMAO plasma levels [331]. In addition, TMAO is absent in germ-free mice and greatly reduced in mice treated with broad-spectrum antibiotics [329, 334]. Therefore, TMAO is a prognostic marker of atherosclerosis that can be modulated via diet and the intestinal microbiota.

While TMAO is strongly correlated with atherosclerosis, determining whether it plays a direct role in causing disease required experiments in atherosclerosis mouse models. Chronic dietary L-carnitine supplementation in mice changes intestinal microbial composition, markedly increases serum TMAO, and worsens atherosclerosis. This does not occur if the intestinal microbiota is concurrently suppressed by antibiotics. In atherosclerosis-prone apolipoprotein ApoE$^{-/-}$ mice, disease is exacerbated by directly adding TMAO to their feed [328]. Importantly, cholesterol, triglycerides, lipoproteins, glucose levels, and hepatic triglyceride plasma levels are not increased in TMAO-fed mice compared to controls. Therefore, in ApoE$^{-/-}$ mice, TMAO is proatherogenic and sufficient to exacerbate atherosclerosis. When intestinal microbiota were isolated from mouse strains with either high or low serum TMAO and transplanted into mice pretreated with antibiotics or germ-free mice, only the microbiota from high TMAO mice were able to exacerbate atherosclerosis and other cardiovascular disease-related phenotypes [333, 335]. These important findings demonstrated that atherosclerosis susceptibility can be transmitted and that TMAO is not only a strong prognostic marker for human cardiovascular disease risk but is also a contributory factor in the pathogenesis of atherosclerotic disease.

2.4.3 Clonal Hematopoiesis of Indeterminate Potential

Hematological cancers are associated with recurrent somatic mutations in specific genes. Recently, somatic mutations were detected in the blood cells of individuals who had no hematologic abnormalities [336, 337]. The most frequent mutations caused loss of function in genes encoding epigenetic regulators (*TET2*, *DNMT3A*, and *ASXL1*) and conferred these cells a selective growth advantage, leading to clonal expansion [336, 337]. Acquisition of somatic mutations that drive clonal expansion in the absence of any signs of blood cancer was termed "clonal hematopoiesis of indeterminate potential" (CHIP) [338]. In addition to the selective advantage the mutations entail, CHIP may also be enhanced by waning hematopoietic stem cell fitness and "loss of regenerative capacity" associated with, for instance, old age. In this case, declining hematopoietic stem cells produced in the bone marrow would contribute to oligoclonal hematopoiesis simply through attrition.

CHIP is an age-related condition that is found in less than 3% of people under 30 years old but is present in slightly over 20% in individuals ages 60–69 [339]. CHIP is surprisingly associated with an increased risk of all-cause mortality, especially from coronary heart disease [336, 337]. In people over 60, CHIP doubles the risk of coronary heart disease, while younger people (<50 years) with CHIP have a 4 times higher risk of myocardial infarction [336].

Murine models of atherosclerosis have demonstrated a causal role for CHIP in cardiovascular disease. Loss of Tet2 function in all or a subpopulation of hematopoietic cells leads to clonal hematopoiesis and accelerated atherosclerosis development [336, 340]. Tet2-deficient macrophages have elevated expression of several chemokine and cytokine genes [336, 340]. Therefore, in mice, the data strongly indicate that Tet2-driven CHIP exacerbates atherosclerosis through enhanced inflammation.

2.5 Inflammation: Just Another Risk Factor or a Unifying Concept?

A role for inflammation in atherosclerotic plaque development has been around a long time, dating back to the mid-1800s with Virchow [341]. Its presence, macroscopically visible in epicardial coronary arteries in subjects with acute coronary syndrome undergoing surgical revascularization, has been one of the impetuses to our research on pathogenesis of atherosclerosis. This local manifestation at the site of acute coronary occlusion has also been seen by Greek interventional cardiologists who described significantly increased temperatures in acute coronary syndromes at the site of occlusion compared to proximal or distal segments of the same coronary, unaffected branches of the coronary artery system, or in chronic stages of the disease. **We now know that inflammation itself plays a fundamental role in mediating all stages of atherosclerosis including initiation, progression, and ultimately, thrombosis** [342].

C-reactive protein (CRP) is a component of the acute phase response and is used as a marker of general inflammation [343]. In epidemiologic studies, measuring systemic CRP levels with a highly sensitive assay (yielding the so-called high-sensitivity or hsCRP level) seems to accurately predict the risk of adverse cardiovascular events [344–349]. However, studies looking at individuals with genetic variations in the CRP gene that give rise to variation in plasma CRP levels clearly indicate that CRP is not causally involved in the pathogenesis of atherosclerosis [350].

The idea that inflammation underlies atherosclerosis development makes sense in terms of the other previously identified risk factors. Inflammation is commonly associated with many of the atherosclerosis risk factors. For example, both oxidized LDL and crystalline cholesterol activate the NLRP3 inflammasome, resulting in a caspase-1 mediated activation and secretion of pro-inflammatory IL-1 family cytokines [351, 352]. Due to the pro-inflammatory nature of adipose tissue, obesity is associated with elevated levels of systemic inflammation [353]. Inflammation is thought to be involved in the development and pathophysiology of hypertension [354]. Infections, diabetes, CKD, and smoking are also all associated with higher levels of systemic inflammation [355–358]. In mouse models of CHIP, macrophages show elevated expression of several chemokine and pro-inflammatory cytokine genes [336, 340]. Therefore, **inflammation is an underlying phenomenon common to almost all identified risk factors for atherosclerosis and has therefore been proposed to be a viable target for both preventive and therapeutic interventions.**

Statins have other, non-lipid-lowering properties, including anti-inflammatory and antioxidant effects that may contribute to their beneficial effects. The anti-inflammatory action of statins is observed through their effect of lowering the levels of CRP. Untangling the benefits of the lipid-lowering and anti-inflammatory properties of statins has been challenging. In the PROVE-IT and IMPROVE-IT trials, patients who lowered both their LDL cholesterol and hsCRP fared better in terms of recurrent vascular events, as compared to patients who only lowered one of these risk factors [108, 359, 360]. The JUPITER (**J**ustification for the **U**se of Statins in **P**revention: an **I**ntervention **T**rial **E**valuating **R**osuvastatin) trial looked at the effect of statins on individuals with normal LDL cholesterol but elevated hsCRP [361]. The results showed that patients with below-guideline levels of LDL cholesterol with elevated hsCRP were still at high risk for cardiovascular events [362]. The Emerging Risk Factor Collaborators calculated the magnitude of independent risk associated with inflammation was at least as large, if not larger, than that of high blood pressure and cholesterol [345].

The CANTOS (Canakinumab Anti-inflammatory Thrombosis Outcomes Study) trial tested whether reducing inflammation among patients who have had a prior heart attack can reduce the risk of future cardiovascular events [363]. It specifically focused on the inflammatory cytokine interleukin (IL)-1β, which is part of the NLRP3 inflammasome that interacts with cholesterol to induce inflammation. Using a monoclonal antibody that neutralizes IL-1β (canakinumab), they found no change in LDL, but a significant reduction in hsCRP and IL-6. The latter is another inflammatory cytokine that is activated downstream of IL-1β. Patients on canakinumab were about 15% less likely to suffer a heart attack or stroke or die from cardiovascular disease and about 30% less likely to need a stent or cardiac bypass surgery [364]. **Therefore, this study was the first direct evidence that inflammation plays a causative role in atherosclerosis development** [365, 366]. Importantly however, overall mortality was significantly increased in the canakinumab group due to an increase in fatal infections. Consequently, anti-inflammatory strategies must always balance the need for inflammation for proper immune defense and damage repair, with its detrimental effects on atherosclerosis development.

2.6 What Risk Factors Do and Do Not Tell Us

Many persons with atherosclerosis do not have established risk factors [367, 368]. Even with an optimal risk factor profile, the lifetime risk of total cardiovascular disease exceeds 30–40% [368]. At the same time, over 50% of individuals with one or two major risk factors remain free from the disease [368]. This implies that we must be missing something, and maybe newly identified risk factors will lead to novel insights and avenues of research. Importantly, as any good epidemiologist will remind you, risk factors are not necessarily causal factors. For example, draining swamps reduces the incidence of malaria. However, one cannot falsely assume that swamps cause malaria when in fact it is the mosquitoes breeding in swamps that are responsible for malaria transmission [369]. Risk factors also do not explain how and why diseases develop, and they shed little insight into the pathomechanisms underlying disease. Risk factors are more likely to have systemic effects but atherosclerosis itself is a site-specific disease (see Chap. 4). Take, for example, even inflammation: exactly how does inflammation trigger plaque formation? Why does systemic inflammation lead to site-specific disease manifestation? Despite systemic inflammation, why do certain branches or segments of the arterial tree consistently remain free from disease? Indeed, few coronary artery disease patients present with peripheral vascular disease, with the exception of carotid artery stenosis. On the contrary, the majority of individuals undergoing interventions for atherosclerotic lesions in the iliac or femoral arteries will also show coronary disease at varying stages of severity. These differences become even more obvious comparing male and female patients with significantly less peripheral vascular disease in women with coronary artery disease. As we begin to explain our hypothesis of atherosclerosis development, one first needs a full understanding of the architecture of the non-diseased and diseased vasculature. Only then will the site specificity of disease and the effect of risk factors on disease make sense.

References

1. Anitschow NN. Deuxième Conférence Internationale de Pathologie Géographique. Oosthoek; 1935.
2. Keys A, Taylor HL, Blackburn H, et al. Coronary heart disease among minnesota business and professional men followed fifteen years. Circulation. 1963;28:381–95. https://doi.org/10.1161/01.CIR.28.3.381.
3. History of the Framingham Heart Study. In: Framingham Heart Study. http://www.framinghamheartstudy.org/about-fhs/history.php (2017). Accessed 8 Aug 2017.
4. Mahmood SS, Levy D, Vasan RS, Wang TJ. The Framingham Heart Study and the epidemiology of cardiovascular disease: a historical perspective. Lancet (London, England). 2014;383:999–1008. https://doi.org/10.1016/S0140-6736(13)61752-3.
5. Dawber TR, Moore FE, Mann GV. Coronary heart disease in the Framingham Study. Am J Public Health Nations Health. 1957;47:4–24.
6. Kannel WB, Dawber TR, Kagan A, et al. Factors of risk in the development of coronary heart disease—six year follow-up experience. The Framingham Study. Ann Intern Med. 1961;55:33–50.
7. O'Donnell CJ, Elosua R. Cardiovascular risk factors. Insights from Framingham Heart Study. Rev Esp Cardiol. 2008;61:299–310. https://doi.org/10.1016/S1885-5857(08)60118-8.
8. Jousilahti P, Vartiainen E, Tuomilehto J, Puska P. Sex, age, cardiovascular risk factors, and coronary heart disease. Circulation. 1999;99.
9. Meadows TA, Bhatt DL, Cannon CP, et al. Ethnic differences in cardiovascular risks and mortality in atherothrombotic disease: insights from the Reduction of Atherothrombosis for Continued Health (REACH) registry. Mayo Clin Proc. 2011;86:960–7. https://doi.org/10.4065/mcp.2011.0010.
10. Schildkraut JM, Myers RH, Cupples LA, et al. Coronary risk associated with age and sex of parental heart disease in the Framingham Study. Am J Cardiol. 1989;64:555–9.
11. Gaeta G, De Michele M, Cuomo S, et al. Arterial abnormalities in the offspring of patients with premature myocardial infarction. N Engl J Med. 2000;343:840–6. https://doi.org/10.1056/NEJM200009213431203.
12. Slack J, Evans KA. The increased risk of death from ischaemic heart disease in first degree relatives of 121 men and 96 women with ischaemic heart disease. J Med Genet. 1966;3:239–57.
13. Juonala M, Viikari JSA, Räsänen L, et al. Young adults with family history of coronary heart disease have increased arterial vulnerability to metabolic risk factors. Arterioscler Thromb Vasc Biol. 2006;26.
14. Kannel WB, McGee DL. Diabetes and cardiovascular disease. The Framingham Study. JAMA. 1979;241:2035–8.
15. Preis SR, Hwang S-J, Coady S, et al. Trends in all-cause and cardiovascular disease mortality among women and men with and without diabetes mellitus in the Framingham Heart Study, 1950 to 2005. Circulation. 2009;119:1728–35. https://doi.org/10.1161/CIRCULATIONAHA.108.829176.
16. Garcia MJ, McNamara PM, Gordon T, Kannell WB. Morbidity and mortality in diabetics in the Framingham population: sixteen year follow-up study. Diabetes. 1974;23.

17. Kuller LH, Velentgas P, Barzilay J, et al. Diabetes mellitus: subclinical cardiovascular disease and risk of incident cardiovascular disease and all-cause mortality. Arterioscler Thromb Vasc Biol. 2000;20:823–9.

18. Creager MA, Lüscher TF, Cosentino F, Beckman JA. Diabetes and vascular disease: pathophysiology, clinical consequences, and medical therapy: Part I. Circulation. 2003;108:1527–32. https://doi.org/10.1161/01.CIR.0000091257.27563.32.

19. Stamler J, Vaccaro O, Neaton JD, Wentworth D. Diabetes, other risk factors, and 12-yr cardiovascular mortality for men screened in the multiple risk factor intervention trial. Diabetes Care. 1993;16:434–44.

20. American Heart Association Statistics Committee and Stroke Statistics Subcommittee. Heart disease and stroke statistics 2017 At-a-Glance. http://professional.heart.org/idc/groups/ahamah-public/@wcm/@sop/@smd/documents/downloadable/ucm_491265.pdf (2017). Accessed 10 July 2017.

21. Howard BV, Rodriguez BL, Bennett PH, et al. Prevention conference VI: diabetes and cardiovascular disease. Circulation. 2002;105.

22. Chait A, Bornfeldt KE. Diabetes and atherosclerosis: is there a role for hyperglycemia? J Lipid Res. 2009;50(Suppl):S335–9. https://doi.org/10.1194/jlr.R800059-JLR200.

23. Tominaga M, Eguchi H, Manaka H, et al. Impaired glucose tolerance is a risk factor for cardiovascular disease, but not impaired fasting glucose. The Funagata Diabetes study. Diabetes Care. 1999;22:920–4.

24. Foley RN, Parfrey PS, Sarnak MJ. Epidemiology of cardiovascular disease in chronic renal disease. J Am Soc Nephrol. 1998;9:S16–23.

25. Sarnak MJ, Levey AS, Schoolwerth AC, et al. Kidney disease as a risk factor for development of cardiovascular disease: a statement from the American heart association councils on kidney in cardiovascular disease, high blood pressure research, clinical cardiology, and epidemiology and prevention. Circulation. 2003;108:2154–69. https://doi.org/10.1161/01.CIR.0000095676.90936.80.

26. Balla S, Nusair MB, Alpert MA. Risk factors for atherosclerosis in patients with chronic kidney disease: recognition and management. Curr Opin Pharmacol. 2013;13:192–9.

27. Tonelli M, Wiebe N, Culleton B, et al. Chronic kidney disease and mortality risk: a systematic review. J Am Soc Nephrol. 2006;17:2034–47. https://doi.org/10.1681/ASN.2005101085.

28. Culleton BF, Larson MG, Wilson PWF, et al. Cardiovascular disease and mortality in a community-based cohort with mild renal insufficiency. Kidney Int. 1999;56:2214–9. https://doi.org/10.1046/j.1523-1755.1999.00773.x.

29. Go AS, Chertow GM, Fan D, et al. Chronic kidney disease and the risks of death, cardiovascular events, and hospitalization. N Engl J Med. 2004;351:1296–305. https://doi.org/10.1056/NEJMoa041031.

30. Hubert HB, Feinleib M, McNamara PM, Castelli WP. Obesity as an independent risk factor for cardiovascular disease: a 26-year follow-up of participants in the Framingham Heart Study. Circulation. 1983;67:968–77.

31. McGill HC, McMahan CA, Herderick EE, et al. Obesity accelerates the progression of coronary atherosclerosis in young men. Circulation. 2002;105:2712–8.

32. Caleyachetty R, Thomas GN, Toulis KA, et al. Metabolically healthy obese and incident cardiovascular disease events among 3.5 million men and women. J Am Coll Cardiol. 2017;70:1429–37. https://doi.org/10.1016/j.jacc.2017.07.763.

33. Sharma S, Batsis JA, Coutinho T, et al. Normal-weight central obesity and mortality risk in older adults with coronary artery disease. Mayo Clin Proc. 2016;91:343–51. https://doi.org/10.1016/j.mayocp.2015.12.007.

34. Herrera BM, Lindgren CM. The genetics of obesity. Curr Diab Rep. 2010;10:498–505. https://doi.org/10.1007/s11892-010-0153-z.

35. Ekelund L-G, Haskell WL, Johnson JL, et al. Physical fitness as a predictor of cardiovascular mortality in asymptomatic North American men. N Engl J Med. 1988;319:1379–84. https://doi.org/10.1056/NEJM198811243192104.

36. Tanasescu M, Leitzmann MF, Rimm EB, et al. Exercise type and intensity in relation to coronary heart disease in men. JAMA. 2000;288:1994–2000.
37. Kodama S, Saito K, Tanaka S, et al. Cardiorespiratory fitness as a quantitative predictor of all-cause mortality and cardiovascular events in healthy men and women: a meta-analysis. JAMA. 2009;301:2024–35. https://doi.org/10.1001/jama.2009.681.
38. Shah RV, Murthy VL, Colangelo LA, et al. Association of fitness in young adulthood with survival and cardiovascular risk. JAMA Intern Med. 2016;176:87. https://doi.org/10.1001/jamainternmed.2015.6309.
39. Sui X, LaMonte MJ, Laditka JN, et al. Cardiorespiratory fitness and adiposity as mortality predictors in older adults. JAMA. 2007;298:2507–16. https://doi.org/10.1001/jama.298.21.2507.
40. McAuley PA, Kokkinos PF, Oliveira RB, et al. Obesity paradox and cardiorespiratory fitness in 12,417 male veterans aged 40 to 70 years. Mayo Clin Proc. 2010;85:115–21. https://doi.org/10.4065/mcp.2009.0562.
41. Kannel WB, Dawber TR, McGee DL. Perspectives on systolic hypertension. The Framingham Study. Circulation. 1980;61:1179–82.
42. MacMahon S, Peto R, Cutler J, et al. Blood pressure, stroke, and coronary heart disease. Part 1, Prolonged differences in blood pressure: prospective observational studies corrected for the regression dilution bias. Lancet (London, England). 1990;335:765–74.
43. Stamler J, Stamler R, Neaton JD. Blood pressure, systolic and diastolic, and cardiovascular risks. US population data. Arch Intern Med. 1993;153:598–615.
44. Kannel WB. Blood pressure as a cardiovascular risk factor: prevention and treatment. JAMA. 1996;275:1571–6.
45. Lakka TA, Salonen R, Kaplan GA, Salonen JT. Blood pressure and the progression of carotid atherosclerosis in middle-aged men. Hypertens. 1999;34:51–6. (Dallas, Tex 1979).
46. Five-year findings of the hypertension detection and follow-up program. I. Reduction in mortality of persons with high blood pressure, including mild hypertension. JAMA. 1979;277:157–66 (Hypertension Detection and Follow-up Program Cooperative Group, 1997).
47. Collins R, Peto R, MacMahon S, et al. Blood pressure, stroke, and coronary heart disease. Part 2, Short-term reductions in blood pressure: overview of randomised drug trials in their epidemiological context. Lancet (London, England). 1990;335:827–38.
48. Prevention of stroke by antihypertensive drug treatment in older persons with isolated systolic hypertension. Final results of the Systolic Hypertension in the Elderly Program (SHEP). JAMA. 1991;265:3255–64 (SHEP Cooperative Research Group).
49. Hansson L, Zanchetti A, Carruthers SG, et al. Effects of intensive blood-pressure lowering and low-dose aspirin in patients with hypertension: principal results of the Hypertension Optimal Treatment (HOT) randomised trial. HOT Study Group. Lancet (London, England). 1998;351:1755–62.
50. Allen N, Berry JD, Ning H, et al. Impact of blood pressure and blood pressure change during middle age on the remaining lifetime risk for cardiovascular disease: the cardiovascular lifetime risk pooling project. Circulation. 2012;125:37–44. https://doi.org/10.1161/CIRCULATIONAHA.110.002774.
51. Vasan RS, Larson MG, Leip EP, et al. Impact of high-normal blood pressure on the risk of cardiovascular disease. N Engl J Med. 2001;345:1291–7. https://doi.org/10.1056/NEJMoa003417.
52. English JP, Willius FA, Berkson J. Tobacco and coronary disease. JAMA. 1940;115:1327. https://doi.org/10.1001/jama.1940.02810420013004.
53. Hammond EC, Horn D. The relationship between human smoking habits and death rates: a follow-up study of 187,766 men. JAMA. 1954;155:1316–28.
54. Hammond EC, Horn D. Smoking and death rates: report on forty-four months of follow-up of 187,783 men. 2. Death rates by cause. JAMA. 1958;166:1294–308.
55. Doll R, Hill AB. The mortality of doctors in relation to their smoking habits; a preliminary report. Br Med J. 1954;1:1451–5.

56. Doyle JT, Dawber TR, Kannel WB, et al. The relationship of cigarette smoking to coronary heart disease; The second report of the combined experience of the Albany, NY, and Framingham, mass, studies. JAMA. 1964;190:886–90.

57. Howard G, Wagenknecht LE, Burke GL, et al. Cigarette smoking and progression of atherosclerosis: the Atherosclerosis Risk in Communities (ARIC) Study. JAMA. 1998;279:119–24.

58. Ambrose JA, Barua RS. The pathophysiology of cigarette smoking and cardiovascular disease: an update. J Am Coll Cardiol. 2004;43:1731–7.

59. Barnoya J, Glantz SA. Cardiovascular effects of secondhand smoke: nearly as large as smoking. Circulation. 2005;111:2684–98. https://doi.org/10.1161/CIRCULATIONAHA.104.492215.

60. Cizek SM, Bedri S, Talusan P, et al. Risk factors for atherosclerosis and the development of preatherosclerotic intimal hyperplasia. Cardiovasc Pathol. 2007;16:344–50. https://doi.org/10.1016/j.carpath.2007.05.007.

61. Rea TD, Heckbert SR, Kaplan RC, et al. Smoking status and risk for recurrent coronary events after myocardial infarction. Ann Intern Med. 2002;137:494–500.

62. Friedman M, Friedland GW. Medicine's 10 greatest discoveries. New Haven & London: Yale University Press;1998.

63. Gofman JW, Lindgren F. The role of lipids and lipoproteins in atherosclerosis. Science. 1950;111:166–71.

64. Konstantinov IE, Mejevoi N, Anichkov NM. Nikolai N. Anichkov and his theory of atherosclerosis. Texas Hear Inst J. 2006;33:417–23.

65. Gofman JW, Lindgren FT, Elliott H. Ultracentrifugal studies of lipoproteins of human serum. J Biol Chem. 1949;179:973–9.

66. Gofman JW. Serum lipoproteins and the evaluation of atherosclerosis. Ann N Y Acad Sci. 1956;64:590–5.

67. Gofman JW, Jones HB, Lindgren FT, et al. Blood lipids and human atherosclerosis. Circulation. 1950;2:161–78.

68. Kinsell LW, Partridge J, Boling L, et al. Dietary modification of serum cholesterol and phospholipid levels. J Clin Endocrinol Metab. 1952;12:909–13. https://doi.org/10.1210/jcem-12-7-909.

69. Ahrens EH, Blankenhorn DH, Tsaltas TT. Effect on human serum lipids of substituting plant for animal fat in diet. Proc Soc Exp Biol Med. 1954;86:872–8.

70. Smit L, van Duin S. About the seven countries study. In: Online Sci. http://www.sevencountriesstudy.com/about-the-study/ (2016). Accessed 9 May 2017.

71. Keys A. Atherosclerosis: a problem in newer public health. J Mt Sinai Hosp N Y. 1953;20:118–39.

72. Keys A, Anderson JT, Fidanza F, et al. Effects of diet on blood lipids in man. Clin Chem. 1955;1:34.

73. Yerushalmy J, Hilleboe HE. Fat in the diet and mortality from heart disease; a methodologic note. N Y State J Med. 1957;57:2343–54.

74. Jacobs DR, Adachi H, Mulder I, et al. Cigarette smoking and mortality risk: twenty-five-year follow-up of the seven countries study. Arch Intern Med. 1999;159:733–40.

75. van den Hoogen PCW, Feskens EJM, Nagelkerke NJD, et al. The relation between blood pressure and mortality due to coronary heart disease among men in different parts of the world. N Engl J Med. 2000;342:1–8. https://doi.org/10.1056/NEJM200001063420101.

76. Keys A, Aravanis C, Blackburn H, et al. Coronary heart disease: overweight and obesity as risk factors. Ann Intern Med. 1972;77:15–27.

77. Verschuren WM, Jacobs DR, Bloemberg BP, et al. Serum total cholesterol and long-term coronary heart disease mortality in different cultures. Twenty-five-year follow-up of the seven countries study. JAMA. 1995;274:131–6.

78. Blackburn H. On the trail of heart attacks in seven countries. http://sph.umn.edu/site/docs/epi/SPH.SevenCountriesStudy.pdf (1995).

79. Kromhout D, Menotti A, Blackburn H. The seven countries study: a scientific adventure in cardiovascular disease epidemiology. Utrecht; 1994.

80. Harcombe Z. Keys six countries graph; 2017. http://www.zoeharcombe.com/2017/02/keys-six-countries-graph/.

81. Minger D. Rescuing good health from bad science. The truth about ancel keys: we 've all got it wrong; 2011. https://deniseminger.com/2011/12/22/the-truth-about-ancel-keys-weve-all-got-it-wrong/.

82. Anderson KM, Castelli WP, Levy D. Cholesterol and mortality: 30 years of follow-up from the Framingham Study. JAMA. 1987;257:2176–80. https://doi.org/10.1001/jama.1987.03390160062027.

83. Frantz ID, Dawson EA, Ashman PL, et al. Test of effect of lipid lowering by diet on cardiovascular risk. The Minnesota Coronary survey. Arterioscler Thromb Vasc Biol. 1989;9:129–35. https://doi.org/10.1161/01.ATV.9.1.129.

84. O'Connor A. A decades-old study, rediscovered, challenges advice on saturated fat. In: New York Times; 2016. https://well.blogs.nytimes.com/2016/04/13/a-decades-old-study-redis-covered-challenges-advice-on-saturated-fat/. Accessed 19 Sep 2017.

85. Leren P. The Oslo diet-heart study. Eleven-year report. Circulation. 1970;42:935–42.

86. Dayton S, Pearce ML. Diet high in unsaturated fat. A controlled clinical trial. Minn Med. 1969;52:1237–42.

87. Turpeinen O, Karvonen MJ, Pekkarinen M, et al. Dietary prevention of coronary heart disease: the Finnish mental hospital study. Int J Epidemiol. 1979;8:99–118.

88. McMichael J. Fats and atheroma: an inquest. Br Med J. 1979;1:173–5.

89. Oliver MF. Lipid lowering and ischaemic heart disease. Acta Med Scand Suppl. 1981;651:285–93.

90. Ahrens EH. Dietary fats and coronary heart disease: unfinished business. Lancet (London, England). 1979;2:1345–8.

91. Stehbens WE. Coronary heart disease, hypercholesterolemia, and atherosclerosis I. False premises. Exp Mol Pathol. 2001;70:103–19. https://doi.org/10.1006/exmp.2000.2340.

92. Stehbens WE. Coronary heart disease, hypercholesterolemia, and atherosclerosis II. Misrepresented Data. Exp Mol Pathol. 2001;70:120–39. https://doi.org/10.1006/exmp.2000.2339.

93. Stehbens WE. The quality of epidemiological data in coronary heart disease and atherosclerosis. J Clin Epidemiol. 1993;46:1337–46.

94. Steinberg D. Thematic review series: the pathogenesis of atherosclerosis. An interpretive history of the cholesterol controversy: Part I. J Lipid Res. 2004;45:1583–93. https://doi.org/10.1194/jlr.R400003-JLR200.

95. Steinberg D. Lowering blood cholesterol to prevent heart disease. NIH Consensus Development Conference statement. Arterioscler Thromb Vasc Biol. 1985;5:404–12. https://doi.org/10.1161/01.ATV.5.4.404.

96. Cabin HS, Roberts WC. Relation of serum total cholesterol and triglyceride levels to the amount and extent of coronary arterial narrowing by atherosclerotic plaque in coronary heart disease. Quantitative analysis of 2,037 five mm segments of 160 major epicardial coronary arteries in 40 necropsy patients. Am J Med. 1982;73:227–34.

97. Marek Z, Jaegermann K, Ciba T. Atherosclerosis and levels of serum cholesterol in post-mortem investigations. Am Heart J. 1962;63:768–74.

98. Hecht HS, Superko HR, Smith LK, McColgan BP. Relation of coronary artery calcium identified by electron beam tomography to serum lipoprotein levels and implications for treatment. Am J Cardiol. 2001;87:406–12.

99. Nitter-Hauge S, Enge I. Relation between blood lipid levels and angiographically evaluated obstructions in coronary arteries. Br Heart J. 1973;35:791–5.

100. Krishnaswami S, Jose VJ, Joseph G. Lack of correlation between coronary risk factors and CAD severity. Int J Cardiol. 1994;47:37–43.

101. Ravnskov U. Is atherosclerosis caused by high cholesterol? QJM. 2002;95:397–403.

102. Ramsden CE, Zamora D, Majchrzak-Hong S, et al. Re-evaluation of the traditional diet-heart hypothesis: analysis of recovered data from Minnesota Coronary Experiment (1968–73). BMJ. 2016;353:i1246.

103. Ravnskov U, Diamond DM, Hama R, et al. Lack of an association or an inverse association between low-density-lipoprotein cholesterol and mortality in the elderly: a systematic review. BMJ Open. 2016;6:e010401. https://doi.org/10.1136/bmjopen-2015-010401.

104. Scandinavian Simvastatin Survival Study Group. Randomised trial of cholesterol lowering in 4444 patients with coronary heart disease: the Scandinavian Simvastatin Survival Study (4S). Lancet. 1994;344:1383–9. https://doi.org/10.1016/S0140-6736(94)90566-5.

105. Ross SD, Allen IE, Connelly JE, et al. Clinical outcomes in statin treatment trials: a meta-analysis. Arch Intern Med. 1999;159:1793–802.

106. Vrecer M, Turk S, Drinovec J, Mrhar A. Use of statins in primary and secondary prevention of coronary heart disease and ischemic stroke. Meta-analysis of randomized trials. Int J Clin Pharmacol Ther. 2003;41:567–77.

107. LaRosa JC, Grundy SM, Waters DD, et al. Intensive lipid lowering with atorvastatin in patients with stable coronary disease. N Engl J Med. 2005;352:1425–35. https://doi.org/10.1056/NEJMoa050461.

108. Cannon CP, Braunwald E, McCabe CH, et al. Intensive versus moderate lipid lowering with statins after acute coronary syndromes. N Engl J Med. 2004;350:1495–504. https://doi.org/10.1056/NEJMoa040583.

109. De Backer G, Ambrosioni E, Borch-Johnsen K, et al. European guidelines on cardiovascular disease prevention in clinical practice. Third joint task force of european and other societies on cardiovascular disease prevention in clinical practice. Eur Heart J. 2003;24:1601–10.

110. Ray KK, Seshasai SRK, Erqou S, et al. Statins and all-cause mortality in high-risk primary prevention: a meta-analysis of 11 randomized controlled trials involving 65,229 participants. Arch Intern Med. 2010;170:1024–31. https://doi.org/10.1001/archinternmed.2010.182.

111. DuBroff R, de Lorgeril M. Cholesterol confusion and statin controversy. World J Cardiol. 2015;7:404–9. https://doi.org/10.4330/wjc.v7.i7.404.

112. de Lorgeril M, Salen P, Martin JL, et al. Mediterranean dietary pattern in a randomized trial: prolonged survival and possible reduced cancer rate. Arch Intern Med. 1998;158:1181–7.

113. Chiuve SE, Fung TT, Rexrode KM, et al. Adherence to a low-risk, healthy lifestyle and risk of sudden cardiac death among women. JAMA. 2011;306. https://doi.org/10.1001/jama.2011.907.

114. Åkesson A, Larsson SC, Discacciati A, Wolk A. Low-risk diet and lifestyle habits in the primary prevention of myocardial infarction in men: a population-based prospective cohort study. J Am Coll Cardiol. 2014;64:1299–306. https://doi.org/10.1016/j.jacc.2014.06.1190.

115. Roth EM, McKenney JM, Hanotin C, et al. Atorvastatin with or without an antibody to PCSK9 in primary hypercholesterolemia. N Engl J Med. 2012;367:1891–900. https://doi.org/10.1056/NEJMoa1201832.

116. Stein EA, Gipe D, Bergeron J, et al. Effect of a monoclonal antibody to PCSK9, REGN727/SAR236553, to reduce low-density lipoprotein cholesterol in patients with heterozygous familial hypercholesterolaemia on stable statin dose with or without ezetimibe therapy: a phase 2 randomised controlled trial. Lancet (London, England). 2012;380:29–36. https://doi.org/10.1016/S0140-6736(12)60771-5.

117. Stein EA, Mellis S, Yancopoulos GD, et al. Effect of a monoclonal antibody to PCSK9 on LDL cholesterol. N Engl J Med. 2012;366:1108–18. https://doi.org/10.1056/NEJMoa1105803.

118. Fitzgerald K, Frank-Kamenetsky M, Shulga-Morskaya S, et al. Effect of an RNA interference drug on the synthesis of proprotein convertase subtilisin/kexin type 9 (PCSK9) and the concentration of serum LDL cholesterol in healthy volunteers: a randomised, single-blind, placebo-controlled, phase 1 trial. Lancet. 2014;383:60–8. https://doi.org/10.1016/S0140-6736(13)61914-5.

119. Fitzgerald K, White S, Borodovsky A, et al. A highly durable RNAi therapeutic inhibitor of PCSK9. N Engl J Med. 2017;376:41–51. https://doi.org/10.1056/NEJMoa1609243.

120. Narasimhan SD. Beyond statins: new therapeutic frontiers for cardiovascular disease. Cell. 2017;169:971–3. https://doi.org/10.1016/j.cell.2017.05.032.

121. Frothingham C. The relationship between acute infectious diseases and arterial lesions. Arch Int Med. 1911;8:153–62.

122. Klotz O, Manning M. Fatty streaks in the intima of arteries. J Pathol Bacteriol. 1911;16:211–20.

123. Martin H. Considérations générales sur la pathogénie des scléroses dystrophiques. In: Revue de Medecine; 1886. p. 1–26.

124. Thérèse. Etude anatomo-pathologiqueet expérimentale sur les artérites secondaires aux maladies infectieuses. Thèse de Paris; 1893.

125. Simnitzky. Über die Häufigkeit von arteriosklerotischen Veränderungen in der Aorta jugendlicher Individuen. Zeitschrift für Heilkd. 1903;24:177.

126. Wiesel. Die Erkrankungen arterieller Gefässe im Verlaufe akuter Infektionen. Zeitschrift für Heilkd. 1906;27:262.

127. Zinserling. Über anisotrope Verfettung der Arterienintima bei Infektionskrankheiten. Zentralblatt für Allg Pathol. 1913;24:627.

128. Thayer W. On the late effects of typhoid fever on the heart and vessels. Am J Med Sci. 1904;77:391–422.

129. Thayer W, Brush C. The relation of acute infections and arteriosclerosis. JAMA. 1904;43:583–4.

130. Osler W. Diseases of the arteries. In: Osler W, MacCrae T, editors. Modern medicine. Its theory and practice in original contributions by Americans and foreign authors. Philadelphia: Lea & Febiger; 1908. p. 426–47.

131. Faber A. Die Arteriosklerose; ihre pathologische Anatomie, ihre Pathogenese und Ätiologie. Jena: Gustav Fischer; 1912.

132. Ophüls W. Arteriosclerosis cardiovascular disease: their relation to infectious diseases, 1st ed. California: University Press, Standford University; 1921.

133. Gilbert L. Artérites infectieuses expérimentales. Compt rend Soc biol. 1889.

134. Crocq. Contribution a L'étude expérimentale des artérites infectieuses. Arch méd exp. 1894;6:583.

135. Boinet R. Recherches expérimentales sur les aortites. Arch méd exp. 1897;9:902.

136. Klotz. The experimental production of arteriosclerosis. Br Med J. 1906;2:1767.

137. Collins SD. Excess mortality from causes other than influenza and pneumonia during influenza epidemics. Public Heal Reports. 1932;47:2159. https://doi.org/10.2307/4580606.

138. Stocks P. The effect of influenza epidemics on the certified cause of death. Lancet. 1935;226:386–95.

139. Fabricant CG, Fabricant J, Litrenta MM, Minick CR. Virus-induced atherosclerosis. J Exp Med. 1978;148:335–40.

140. Moazed TC, Campbell LA, Rosenfeld ME, et al. Chlamydia pneumoniae infection accelerates the progression of atherosclerosis in apolipoprotein E-deficient mice. J Infect Dis. 1999;180:238–41. https://doi.org/10.1086/314855.

141. Hu H, Pierce GN, Zhong G. The atherogenic effects of chlamydia are dependent on serum cholesterol and specific to Chlamydia pneumoniae. J Clin Invest. 1999;103:747–53. https://doi.org/10.1172/JCI4582.

142. Li L, Messas E, Batista EL, et al. Porphyromonas gingivalis infection accelerates the progression of atherosclerosis in a heterozygous apolipoprotein E-deficient murine model. Circulation. 2002;105:861–7.

143. Jia R, Kurita-Ochiai T, Oguchi S, Yamamoto M. Periodontal pathogen accelerates lipid peroxidation and atherosclerosis. J Dent Res. 2013;92:247–52. https://doi.org/10.1177/0022034513475625.

144. Chen X, Wang J, Wang Y, et al. Helicobacter pylori infection enhances atherosclerosis in high-cholesterol diet fed C57BL/6 mice. Zhonghua Xin Xue Guan Bing Za Zhi. 2010;38:259–63.

145. Hsich E, Zhou YF, Paigen B, et al. Cytomegalovirus infection increases development of atherosclerosis in Apolipoprotein-E knockout mice. Atherosclerosis. 2001;156:23–8.

146. Vliegen I, Herngreen SB, Grauls GELM, et al. Mouse cytomegalovirus antigenic immune stimulation is sufficient to aggravate atherosclerosis in hypercholesterolemic mice. Atherosclerosis. 2005;181:39–44. https://doi.org/10.1016/j.atherosclerosis.2004.12.035.

147. Vliegen I, Duijvestijn A, Grauls G, et al. Cytomegalovirus infection aggravates atherogenesis in apoE knockout mice by both local and systemic immune activation. Microbes Infect. 2004;6:17–24.

148. Rosenfeld ME, Campbell LA. Pathogens and atherosclerosis: update on the potential contribution of multiple infectious organisms to the pathogenesis of atherosclerosis. Thromb Haemost. 2011;106:858–67. https://doi.org/10.1160/TH11-06-0392.

149. Campbell LA, Rosenfeld ME. Infection and atherosclerosis development. Arch Med Res. 2015;46:339–50. https://doi.org/10.1016/j.arcmed.2015.05.006.

150. Sorrentino R, Yilmaz A, Schubert K, et al. A single infection with Chlamydia pneumoniae is sufficient to exacerbate atherosclerosis in ApoE deficient mice. Cell Immunol. 2015;294:25–32. https://doi.org/10.1016/j.cellimm.2015.01.007.

151. Blessing E, Campbell LA, Rosenfeld ME, et al. Chlamydia pneumoniae infection accelerates hyperlipidemia induced atherosclerotic lesion development in C57BL/6 J mice. Atherosclerosis. 2001;158:13–7. https://doi.org/10.1016/S0021-9150(00)00758-9.

152. Ezzahiri R, Nelissen-Vrancken HJMG, Kurvers HAJM, et al. Chlamydophila pneumoniae (Chlamydia pneumoniae) accelerates the formation of complex atherosclerotic lesions in Apo E3-Leiden mice. Cardiovasc Res. 2002;56:269–76.

153. Muhlestein JB. Chlamydia pneumoniae—Induced atherosclerosis in a rabbit model. J Infect Dis. 2000;181:S505–7. https://doi.org/10.1086/315627.

154. Haidari M, Wyde PR, Litovsky S, et al. Influenza virus directly infects, inflames, and resides in the arteries of atherosclerotic and normal mice. Atherosclerosis. 2010;208:90–6. https://doi.org/10.1016/j.atherosclerosis.2009.07.028.

155. Naghavi M, Wyde P, Litovsky S, et al. Influenza infection exerts prominent inflammatory and thrombotic effects on the atherosclerotic plaques of apolipoprotein E-deficient mice. Circulation. 2003;107:762–8.

156. Jain A, Batista EL, Serhan C, et al. Role for periodontitis in the progression of lipid deposition in an animal model. Infect Immun. 2003;71:6012–8.

157. Lalla E, Lamster IB, Hofmann MA, et al. Oral infection with a periodontal pathogen accelerates early atherosclerosis in apolipoprotein E-null mice. Arterioscler Thromb Vasc Biol. 2003;23:1405–11. https://doi.org/10.1161/01.ATV.0000082462.26258.FE.

158. Watson C, Alp NJ. Role of Chlamydia pneumoniae in atherosclerosis. Clin Sci (Lond). 2008;114:509–31. https://doi.org/10.1042/CS20070298.

159. Al-Ghamdi A, Jiman-Fatani AA, El-Banna H. Role of Chlamydia pneumoniae, Helicobacter pylori and cytomegalovirus in coronary artery disease. Pak J Pharm Sci. 2011;24:95–101.

160. Boman J, Hammerschlag MR. Chlamydia pneumoniae and atherosclerosis: critical assessment of diagnostic methods and relevance to treatment studies. Clin Microbiol Rev. 2002;15:1–20.

161. Saikku P, Leinonen M, Mattila K, et al. Serological evidence of an association of a novel Chlamydia, TWAR, with chronic coronary heart disease and acute myocardial infarction. Lancet (London, England). 1988;2:983–6.

162. Jha HC, Prasad J, Mittal A. High immunoglobulin A seropositivity for combined Chlamydia pneumoniae, Helicobacter pylori infection, and high-sensitivity C-reactive protein in coronary artery disease patients in India can serve as atherosclerotic marker. Heart Vessels. 2008;23:390–6. https://doi.org/10.1007/s00380-008-1062-9.

163. Filardo S, Di Pietro M, Farcomeni A, et al. Chlamydia pneumoniae-mediated inflammation in atherosclerosis: a meta-analysis. Mediat Inflamm. 2015;2015:1–9. https://doi.org/10.1155/2015/378658.

164. Park MJ, Choi SH, Kim D, et al. Association between Helicobacter pylori seropositivity and the coronary artery calcium score in a screening population. Gut Liver. 2011;5:321–7. https://doi.org/10.5009/gnl.2011.5.3.321.

165. Nieto FJ, Adam E, Sorlie P, et al. Cohort study of cytomegalovirus infection as a risk factor for carotid intimal-medial thickening, a measure of subclinical atherosclerosis. Circulation. 1996;94:922–7.

166. Bloemenkamp DGM, Mali WPTM, Visseren FLJ, van der Graaf Y. Meta-analysis of sero-epidemiologic studies of the relation between Chlamydia pneumoniae and atherosclerosis: does study design influence results? Am Heart J. 2003;145:409–17. https://doi.org/10.1067/mhj.2003.20.

167. Longo-Mbenza B, Nkondi M, et al. Helicobacter pylori infection is identified as a cardiovascular risk factor in Central Africans. Vasc Health Risk Manag. 2012;6:455. https://doi.org/10.2147/VHRM.S28680.

168. Roberts ET, Haan MN, Dowd JB, Aiello AE. Cytomegalovirus antibody levels, inflammation, and mortality among elderly Latinos over 9 years of follow-up. Am J Epidemiol. 2010;172:363–71. https://doi.org/10.1093/aje/kwq177.

169. Tamer GS, Tengiz I, Ercan E, et al. Helicobacter pylori seropositivity in patients with acute coronary syndromes. Dig Dis Sci. 2009;54:1253–6. https://doi.org/10.1007/s10620-008-0482-9.

170. Folsom AR, Nieto FJ, Sorlie P, et al. Helicobacter pylori seropositivity and coronary heart disease incidence. Atherosclerosis Risk In Communities (ARIC) study investigators. Circulation. 1998;98:845–50.

171. Ozdogru I, Kalay N, Dogan A, et al. The relationship between Helicobacter pylori IgG titre and coronary atherosclerosis. Acta Cardiol. 2007;62:501–5. https://doi.org/10.2143/AC.62.5.2023414.

172. Danesh J, Whincup P, Walker M, et al. Chlamydia pneumoniae IgG titres and coronary heart disease: prospective study and meta-analysis. BMJ. 2000;321:208–13.

173. Spodick DH, Flessas AP, Johnson MM. Association of acute respiratory symptoms with onset of acute myocardial infarction: prospective investigation of 150 consecutive patients and matched control patients. Am J Cardiol. 1984;53:481–2.

174. Penttinen J, Valonen P. The risk of myocardial infarction among Finnish farmers seeking medical care for an infection. Am J Public Health. 1996;86:1440–2.

175. Spencer FA, Goldberg RJ, Becker RC, Gore JM. Seasonal distribution of acute myocardial infarction in the second National Registry of Myocardial Infarction. J Am Coll Cardiol. 1998;31:1226–33.

176. Sheth T, Nair C, Muller J, Yusuf S. Increased winter mortality from acute myocardial infarction and stroke: the effect of age. J Am Coll Cardiol. 1999;33:1916–9. https://doi.org/10.1016/s0735-1097(99)00137-0.

177. Barnes M, Heywood AE, Mahimbo A, et al. Acute myocardial infarction and influenza: a meta-analysis of case-control studies. Heart. 2015;101:1738–47. https://doi.org/10.1136/heartjnl-2015-307691.

178. Vlachopoulos CV, Terentes-Printzios DG, Aznaouridis KA, et al. Association between pneumococcal vaccination and cardiovascular outcomes: a systematic review and meta-analysis of cohort studies. Eur J Prev Cardiol. 2015;22:1185–99. https://doi.org/10.1177/2047487314549512.

179. Fountoulaki K, Tsiodras S, Polyzogopoulou E, et al. Beneficial effects of vaccination on cardiovascular events: myocardial infarction, stroke, heart failure. Cardiology. 2018;141:98–106. https://doi.org/10.1159/000493572.

180. Naghavi M, Barlas Z, Siadaty S, et al. Association of influenza vaccination and reduced risk of recurrent myocardial infarction. Circulation. 2000;102:3039–45.

181. Siscovick DS, Raghunathan TE, Lin D, et al. Influenza vaccination and the risk of primary cardiac arrest. Am J Epidemiol. 2000;152:674–7.

182. Xu Y, Wang Q, Liu Y, et al. Association between Helicobacter pylori infection and carotid atherosclerosis in patients with vascular dementia. J Neurol Sci. 2016;362:73–7. https://doi.org/10.1016/j.jns.2016.01.025.

183. Pietroiusti A, Diomedi M, Silvestrini M, et al. Cytotoxin-associated gene-A–positive Helicobacter pylori strains are associated with atherosclerotic stroke. Circulation. 2002;106:580–4.

184. Diomedi M, Pietroiusti A, Silvestrini M, et al. CagA-positive Helicobacter pylori strains may influence the natural history of atherosclerotic stroke. Neurology. 2004;63:800–4.

185. Sun J, Rangan P, Bhat SS, Liu L. A meta-analysis of the association between Helicobacter pylori infection and risk of coronary heart disease from published prospective studies. Helicobacter. 2016;21:11–23. https://doi.org/10.1111/hel.12234.

186. Mendall MA, Goggin PM, Molineaux N, et al. Relation of Helicobacter pylori infection and coronary heart disease. Br Heart J. 1994;71:437–9.

187. Shmuely H, Wattad M, Solodky A, et al. Association of Helicobacter pylori with coronary artery disease and myocardial infarction assessed by myocardial perfusion imaging. Isr Med Assoc J. 2014;16:341–6.

188. Lockhart PB, Bolger AF, Papapanou PN, et al. Periodontal disease and atherosclerotic vascular disease: does the evidence support an independent association?: a scientific statement from the American Heart Association. Circulation. 2012;125:2520–44. https://doi.org/10.1161/CIR.0b013e31825719f3.

189. Trevisan M, Dorn J. The relationship between periodontal disease (pd) and cardiovascular disease (cvd). Mediterr J Hematol Infect Dis. 2010;2:e2010030. https://doi.org/10.4084/MJHID.2010.030.

190. Mattila KJ, Nieminen MS, Valtonen VV, et al. Association between dental health and acute myocardial infarction. BMJ. 1989;298:779–81.

191. de Oliveira C, Watt R, Hamer M. Toothbrushing, inflammation, and risk of cardiovascular disease: results from Scottish Health Survey. BMJ. 2010;340:c2451.

192. Amar S, Al-Hashemi J. Periodontal innate immune mechanisms relevant to atherosclerosis. In: Vascular responses to pathogens. NIH Public Access; 2015, p. 75–85.

193. Tang K, Lin M, Wu Y, Yan F. Alterations of serum lipid and inflammatory cytokine profiles in patients with coronary heart disease and chronic periodontitis: a pilot study. J Int Med Res. 2011;39:238–48. https://doi.org/10.1177/147323001103900126.

194. Hansen GM, Egeberg A, Holmstrup P, Hansen PR. Relation of periodontitis to risk of cardiovascular and all-cause mortality (from a Danish nationwide cohort study). Am J Cardiol. 2016;118:489–93. https://doi.org/10.1016/j.amjcard.2016.05.036.

195. Beukers NGFM, van der Heijden GJMG, van Wijk AJ, Loos BG. Periodontitis is an independent risk indicator for atherosclerotic cardiovascular diseases among 60,174 participants in a large dental school in the Netherlands. J Epidemiol Community Health. 2017;71:37–42. https://doi.org/10.1136/jech-2015-206745.

196. Piconi S, Trabattoni D, Luraghi C, et al. Treatment of periodontal disease results in improvements in endothelial dysfunction and reduction of the carotid intima-media thickness. FASEB J. 2009;23:1196–204. https://doi.org/10.1096/fj.08-119578.

197. Toregeani JF, Nassar CA, Nassar PO, et al. Evaluation of periodontitis treatment effects on carotid intima-media thickness and expression of laboratory markers related to atherosclerosis. Gen Dent. 2016;64:55–62.

198. Orlandi M, Suvan J, Petrie A, et al. Association between periodontal disease and its treatment, flow-mediated dilatation and carotid intima-media thickness: a systematic review and meta-analysis. Atherosclerosis. 2014;236:39–46. https://doi.org/10.1016/j.atherosclerosis.2014.06.002.

199. Eberhard J, Grote K, Luchtefeld M, et al. Experimental gingivitis induces systemic inflammatory markers in young healthy individuals: a single-subject interventional study. PLoS One. 2013;8:e55265. https://doi.org/10.1371/journal.pone.0055265.

200. Ameriso SF, Fridman EA, Leiguarda RC, Sevlever GE. Detection of Helicobacter pylori in human carotid atherosclerotic plaques. Stroke. 2001;32:385–91.
201. Ramirez JA. Isolation of Chlamydia pneumoniae from the coronary artery of a patient with coronary atherosclerosis. The Chlamydia pneumoniae/Atherosclerosis Study Group. Ann Intern Med. 1996;125:979–82.
202. Kuo CC, Gown AM, Benditt EP, Grayston JT. Detection of Chlamydia pneumoniae in aortic lesions of atherosclerosis by immunocytochemical stain. Arterioscler Thromb J Vasc Biol. 1993;13:1501–4.
203. Izadi M, Fazel M, Saadat SH, et al. Cytomegalovirus localization in atherosclerotic plaques is associated with acute coronary syndromes: report of 105 patients. Methodist Debakey Cardiovasc J. 2012;8:42–6.
204. Kaplan M, Yavuz SS, Cinar B, et al. Detection of Chlamydia pneumoniae and Helicobacter pylori in atherosclerotic plaques of carotid artery by polymerase chain reaction. Int J Infect Dis. 2006;10:116–23. https://doi.org/10.1016/j.ijid.2004.10.008.
205. Kalayoglu MV, Libby P, Byrne GI. Chlamydia pneumoniae as an emerging risk factor in cardiovascular disease. JAMA. 2002;288:2724–31.
206. Kilic A, Onguru O, Tugcu H, et al. Detection of cytomegalovirus and Helicobacter pylori DNA in arterial walls with grade III atherosclerosis by PCR. Polish J Microbiol. 2006;55:333–7.
207. Shor A, Phillips JI, Ong G, et al. Chlamydia pneumoniae in atheroma: consideration of criteria for causality. J Clin Pathol. 1998;51:812–7.
208. Sessa R, Di Pietro M, Schiavoni G, et al. Chlamydia pneumoniae DNA in patients with symptomatic carotid atherosclerotic disease. J Vasc Surg. 2003;37:1027–31. https://doi.org/10.1067/mva.2003.200.
209. Jackson LA, Campbell LA, Kuo CC, et al. Isolation of Chlamydia pneumoniae from a carotid endarterectomy specimen. J Infect Dis. 1997;176:292–5.
210. Maass M, Bartels C, Engel PM, et al. Endovascular presence of viable Chlamydia pneumoniae is a common phenomenon in coronary artery disease. J Am Coll Cardiol. 1998;31:827–32.
211. Rafferty B, Dolgilevich S, Kalachikov S, et al. Cultivation of Enterobacter hormaechei from human atherosclerotic tissue. J Atheroscler Thromb. 2011;18:72–81.
212. Farsak B, Yildirir A, Akyön Y, et al. Detection of Chlamydia pneumoniae and Helicobacter pylori DNA in human atherosclerotic plaques by PCR. J Clin Microbiol. 2000;38:4408–11.
213. Melnick JL, Hu C, Burek J, et al. Cytomegalovirus DNA in arterial walls of patients with atherosclerosis. J Med Virol. 1994;42:170–4.
214. Kozarov EV, Dorn BR, Shelburne CE, et al. Human atherosclerotic plaque contains viable invasive Actinobacillus actinomycetemcomitans and Porphyromonas gingivalis. Arterioscler Thromb Vasc Biol. 2005;25:e17–8. https://doi.org/10.1161/01.ATV.0000155018.67835.1a.
215. Shanmugam NP, Harrison PM, Devlin J, et al. Selective use of endoscopic retrograde cholangiopancreatography in the diagnosis of biliary atresia in infants younger than 100 days. J Pediatr Gastroenterol Nutr. 2009;49:435–41. https://doi.org/10.1097/MPG.0b013e3181a8711f.
216. Haraszthy VI, Zambon JJ, Trevisan M, et al. Identification of periodontal pathogens in atheromatous plaques. J Periodontol. 2000;71:1554–60. https://doi.org/10.1902/jop.2000.71.10.1554.
217. Serra e Silva Filho W, Casarin RCV, Nicolela EL, et al. Microbial diversity similarities in periodontal pockets and atheromatous plaques of cardiovascular disease patients. PLoS One. 2014;9:e109761. https://doi.org/10.1371/journal.pone.0109761.
218. Chhibber-Goel J, Singhal V, Bhowmik D, et al. Linkages between oral commensal bacteria and atherosclerotic plaques in coronary artery disease patients. NPJ Biofilms Microbiomes. 2016;2:7. https://doi.org/10.1038/s41522-016-0009-7.

219. Koren O, Spor A, Felin J, et al. Human oral, gut, and plaque microbiota in patients with atherosclerosis. Proc Natl Acad Sci USA. 2011;108(Suppl):4592–8. https://doi.org/10.1073/pnas.1011383107.

220. Eberhard J, Stumpp N, Winkel A, et al. Streptococcus mitis and Gemella haemolysans were simultaneously found in atherosclerotic and oral plaques of elderly without periodontitis-a pilot study. Clin Oral Investig. 2017;21:447–52. https://doi.org/10.1007/s00784-016-1811-6.

221. Renko J, Lepp PW, Oksala N, et al. Bacterial signatures in atherosclerotic lesions represent human commensals and pathogens. Atherosclerosis. 2008;201:192–7. https://doi.org/10.1016/j.atherosclerosis.2008.01.006.

222. Calandrini CA, Ribeiro AC, Gonnelli AC, et al. Microbial composition of atherosclerotic plaques. Oral Dis. 2014;20:e128–34. https://doi.org/10.1111/odi.12205.

223. Mitra S, Drautz-Moses DI, Alhede M, et al. In silico analyses of metagenomes from human atherosclerotic plaque samples. Microbiome. 2015;3:38. https://doi.org/10.1186/s40168-015-0100-y.

224. Armingohar Z, Jørgensen JJ, Kristoffersen AK, et al. Bacteria and bacterial DNA in atherosclerotic plaque and aneurysmal wall biopsies from patients with and without periodontitis. J Oral Microbiol. 2014;6. https://doi.org/10.3402/jom.v6.23408.

225. Prasad A, Zhu J, Halcox JPJ, et al. Predisposition to atherosclerosis by infections: role of endothelial dysfunction. Circulation. 2002;106:184–90.

226. Espinola-Klein C, Rupprecht HJ, Blankenberg S, et al. Impact of infectious burden on extent and long-term prognosis of atherosclerosis. Circulation. 2002;105:15–21. https://doi.org/10.1161/hc0102.101362.

227. Espinola-Klein C, Rupprecht HJ, Blankenberg S, et al. Impact of infectious burden on progression of carotid atherosclerosis. Stroke. 2002;33:2581–6. https://doi.org/10.1161/01.STR.0000034789.82859.A4.

228. Elkind MSV, Luna JM, Moon YP, et al. Infectious burden and carotid plaque thickness: the northern Manhattan study. Stroke. 2010;41. https://doi.org/10.1161/STROKEAHA.109.571299.

229. Grayston JT. Antibiotic treatment of atherosclerotic cardiovascular disease. Circulation. 2003;107:1228–30.

230. Gupta S, Leatham EW, Carrington D, et al. Elevated Chlamydia pneumoniae antibodies, cardiovascular events, and azithromycin in male survivors of myocardial infarction. Circulation. 1997;96:404–7.

231. Kowalski M. Helicobacter pylori (H. pylori) infection in coronary artery disease: influence of H. pylori eradication on coronary artery lumen after percutaneous transluminal coronary angioplasty. The detection of H. pylori specific DNA in human coronary atherosclerotic plaque. J Physiol Pharmacol. 2001;52:3–31.

232. Blum A, Tamir S, Mualem K, et al. Endothelial dysfunction is reversible in Helicobacter pylori-positive subjects. Am J Med. 2011;124:1171–4. https://doi.org/10.1016/j.amjmed.2011.08.015.

233. Wu Y, Tao Z, Song C, et al. Overexpression of YKL-40 predicts plaque instability in carotid atherosclerosis with CagA-positive Helicobacter Pylori infection. PLoS One. 2013;8:e59996. https://doi.org/10.1371/journal.pone.0059996.

234. Nazligul Y, Aslan M, Horoz M, et al. The effect on serum myeloperoxidase activity and oxidative status of eradication treatment in patients Helicobacter pylori infected. Clin Biochem. 2011;44:647–9. https://doi.org/10.1016/j.clinbiochem.2011.03.001.

235. Kebapcilar L, Sari I, Renkal AH, et al. The influence of Helicobacter pylori eradication on leptin, soluble CD40 ligand, oxidative stress and body composition in patients with peptic ulcer disease. Intern Med. 2009;48:2055–9.

236. O'Connor CM, Dunne MW, Pfeffer MA, et al. Azithromycin for the secondary prevention of coronary heart disease events: the WIZARD study: a randomized controlled trial. JAMA. 2003;290:1459–66. https://doi.org/10.1001/jama.290.11.1459.

237. Grayston JT, Kronmal RA, Jackson LA, et al. Azithromycin for the secondary prevention of coronary events. N Engl J Med. 2005;352:1637–45. https://doi.org/10.1056/NEJMoa043526.
238. Jespersen CM, Als-Nielsen B, Damgaard M, et al. Randomised placebo controlled multicentre trial to assess short term clarithromycin for patients with stable coronary heart disease: CLARICOR trial. BMJ. 2006;332:22–7. https://doi.org/10.1136/bmj.38666.653600.55.
239. Song Z, Brassard P, Brophy JM. A meta-analysis of antibiotic use for the secondary prevention of cardiovascular diseases. Can J Cardiol. 2008;24:391–5.
240. Grayston JT, Belland RJ, Byrne GI, et al. Infection with Chlamydia pneumoniae as a cause of coronary heart disease: the hypothesis is still untested. Pathog Dis. 2015;73:1–9. https://doi.org/10.1093/femspd/ftu015.
241. Campbell LA, Rosenfeld ME. Persistent C. pneumoniae infection in atherosclerotic lesions: rethinking the clinical trials. Front Cell Infect Microbiol. 2014;4:1–4. https://doi.org/10.3389/fcimb.2014.00034.
242. Kuck K-H, Eggebrecht H, Figulla HR, et al. Qualitätskriterien zur Durchführung der transvaskulären Aortenklappenimplantation (TAVI). DGK. 2015;9:11–26. https://doi.org/10.1007/s12181-014-0622-8.
243. Zagari RM, Rabitti S, Eusebi LH, Bazzoli F. Treatment of Helicobacter pylori infection: a clinical practice update. Eur J Clin Invest. 2017. https://doi.org/10.1111/eci.12857.
244. Kim SY, Choi DJ, Chung J-W. Antibiotic treatment for Helicobacter pylori: is the end coming? World J Gastrointest Pharmacol Ther. 2015;6:183–98. https://doi.org/10.4292/wjgpt.v6.i4.183.
245. Schlesselman L. Novel risk factors for atherosclerotic disease. http://www.medscape.org/viewarticle/418378 (2001). Accessed 9 May 2017.
246. Fruchart J-C. New risk factors for atherosclerosis and patient risk assessment. Circulation. 2004;109:III-15–III-19. https://doi.org/10.1161/01.CIR.0000131513.33892.5b.
247. McCully KS. Chemical pathology of homocysteine. I. Atherogenesis. Ann Clin Lab Sci. 1993;23:477–93.
248. McCully KS. Homocysteine and the pathogenesis of atherosclerosis. Expert Rev Clin Pharmacol. 2015;8:211–9. https://doi.org/10.1586/17512433.2015.1010516.
249. Smulders YM, Blom HJ. The homocysteine controversy. J Inherit Metab Dis. 2011;34:93–9. https://doi.org/10.1007/s10545-010-9151-1.
250. Martí-Carvajal AJ, Solà I, Lathyris D, Dayer M. Homocysteine-lowering interventions for preventing cardiovascular events. Cochrane Database Syst Rev. 2017;8:CD006612. https://doi.org/10.1002/14651858.CD006612.pub5.
251. Miller ER, Juraschek S, Pastor-Barriuso R, et al. Meta-analysis of folic acid supplementation trials on risk of cardiovascular disease and risk interaction with baseline homocysteine levels. Am J Cardiol. 2010;106:517–27. https://doi.org/10.1016/j.amjcard.2010.03.064.
252. Effects of homocysteine-lowering with folic acid plus vitamin B12 vs placebo on mortality and major morbidity in myocardial infarction survivors. JAMA. 2010;303:2486. https://doi.org/10.1001/jama.2010.840.
253. Bønaa KH, Njølstad I, Ueland PM, et al. Homocysteine lowering and cardiovascular events after acute myocardial infarction. N Engl J Med. 2006;354:1578–88. https://doi.org/10.1056/NEJMoa055227.
254. Lonn E, Yusuf S, Arnold MJ, et al. Homocysteine lowering with folic acid and B vitamins in vascular disease. N Engl J Med. 2006;354:1567–77. https://doi.org/10.1056/NEJMoa060900.
255. Jamison RL, Hartigan P, Kaufman JS, et al. Effect of homocysteine lowering on mortality and vascular disease in advanced chronic kidney disease and end-stage renal disease: a randomized controlled trial. JAMA. 2007;298:1163–70. https://doi.org/10.1001/jama.298.10.1163.

256. Miller MR, Shaw CA, Langrish JP. From particles to patients: oxidative stress and the cardiovascular effects of air pollution. Future Cardiol. 2012;8:577–602. https://doi.org/10.2217/fca.12.43.

257. WHO | Ambient air pollution. In: WHO. http://www.who.int/gho/phe/outdoor_air_pollution/en/ (2016). Accessed 10 Oct 2017.

258. Donaldson K, Stone V, Clouter A, et al. Ultrafine particles. Occup Environ Med. 2001;58(211–6):199.

259. Cosselman KE, Navas-Acien A, Kaufman JD. Environmental factors in cardiovascular disease. Nat Rev Cardiol. 2015;12:627–42. https://doi.org/10.1038/nrcardio.2015.152.

260. US EPA National Center for Environmental Assessment, Research Triangle Park Nc EMAG, Sacks J. Integrated Science Assessment (ISA) for particulate matter (Final Report, Dec 2009); 2009. https://cfpub.epa.gov/ncea/risk/recordisplay.cfm?deid=216546. Accessed 10 Oct 2017.

261. WHO | Air quality guidelines-global update 2005. In: WHO; 2011. http://www.who.int/phe/health_topics/outdoorair/outdoorair_aqg/en/. Accessed 10 Oct 2017.

262. Cohen AJ, Brauer M, Burnett R, et al. Estimates and 25-year trends of the global burden of disease attributable to ambient air pollution: an analysis of data from the Global Burden of Diseases Study 2015. Lancet. 2017;389:1907–18. https://doi.org/10.1016/S0140-6736(17)30505-6.

263. Dockery DW, Pope CA, Xu X, et al. An association between air pollution and mortality in six U.S. Cities. N Engl J Med. 1993;329:1753–9. https://doi.org/10.1056/NEJM199312093292401.

264. Pope CA, Thun MJ, Namboodiri MM, et al. Particulate air pollution as a predictor of mortality in a prospective study of U.S. adults. Am J Respir Crit Care Med. 1995;151:669–74. https://doi.org/10.1164/ajrccm/151.3_Pt_1.669.

265. Hoek G, Brunekreef B, Goldbohm S, et al. Association between mortality and indicators of traffic-related air pollution in the Netherlands: a cohort study. Lancet. 2002;360:1203–9. https://doi.org/10.1016/S0140-6736(02)11280-3.

266. Beelen R, Stafoggia M, Raaschou-Nielsen O, et al. Long-term exposure to air pollution and cardiovascular mortality: an analysis of 22 European cohorts. Epidemiology. 2014;25:368–78. https://doi.org/10.1097/EDE.0000000000000076.

267. Vedal S, Campen MJ, McDonald JD, et al. National Particle Component Toxicity (NPACT) initiative report on cardiovascular effects. Res Rep Health Eff Inst. 2013:5–8.

268. Beelen R, Raaschou-Nielsen O, Stafoggia M, et al. Effects of long-term exposure to air pollution on natural-cause mortality: an analysis of 22 European cohorts within the multicentre ESCAPE project. Lancet. 2014;383:785–95. https://doi.org/10.1016/S0140-6736(13)62158-3.

269. Samet JM, Dominici F, Curriero FC, et al. Fine particulate air pollution and mortality in 20 U.S. cities, 1987–1994. N Engl J Med. 2000;343:1742–9. https://doi.org/10.1056/NEJM200012143432401.

270. Katsouyanni K, Touloumi G, Spix C, et al. Short-term effects of ambient sulphur dioxide and particulate matter on mortality in 12 European cities: results from time series data from the APHEA project. Air pollution and health: a european approach. BMJ. 1997;314:1658–63.

271. Katsouyanni K, Touloumi G, Samoli E, et al. Confounding and effect modification in the short-term effects of ambient particles on total mortality: results from 29 European cities within the APHEA2 project. Epidemiology. 2001;12:521–31.

272. Pope CA, Turner MC, Burnett RT, et al. Relationships between fine particulate air pollution, cardiometabolic disorders, and cardiovascular mortality. Circ Res. 2015;116:108–15. https://doi.org/10.1161/CIRCRESAHA.116.305060.

273. Hartiala J, Breton CV, Tang WHW, et al. Ambient air pollution is associated with the severity of coronary atherosclerosis and incident myocardial infarction in patients undergoing elective cardiac evaluation. J Am Heart Assoc. 2016;5:e003947. https://doi.org/10.1161/JAHA.116.003947.

274. Cesaroni G, Forastiere F, Stafoggia M, et al. Long term exposure to ambient air pollution and incidence of acute coronary events: prospective cohort study and meta-analysis in 11 European cohorts from the ESCAPE project. BMJ. 2014;348:f7412. https://doi.org/10.1136/bmj.f7412.

275. Miller KA, Siscovick DS, Sheppard L, et al. Long-term exposure to air pollution and incidence of cardiovascular events in women. N Engl J Med. 2007;356:447–58. https://doi.org/10.1056/NEJMoa054409.

276. Newby DE, Mannucci PM, Tell GS, et al. Expert position paper on air pollution and cardiovascular disease. Eur Heart J. 2015;36:83–93. https://doi.org/10.1093/eurheartj/ehu458.

277. Adar SD, Sheppard L, Vedal S, et al. Fine particulate air pollution and the progression of carotid intima-medial thickness: a prospective cohort study from the multi-ethnic study of atherosclerosis and air pollution. PLoS Med. 2013;10:e1001430. https://doi.org/10.1371/journal.pmed.1001430.

278. Akintoye E, Shi L, Obaitan I, et al. Association between fine particulate matter exposure and subclinical atherosclerosis: a meta-analysis. Eur J Prev Cardiol. 2016;23:602–12. https://doi.org/10.1177/2047487315588758.

279. Provost EB, Madhloum N, Int Panis L, et al. Carotid intima-media thickness, a marker of subclinical atherosclerosis, and particulate air pollution exposure: the meta-analytical evidence. PLoS One. 2015;10:e0127014. https://doi.org/10.1371/journal.pone.0127014.

280. Dorans KS, Wilker EH, Li W, et al. Residential proximity to major roads, exposure to fine particulate matter, and coronary artery calcium: the Framingham Heart Study. Arterioscler Thromb Vasc Biol. 2016;36:1679–85. https://doi.org/10.1161/ATVBAHA.116.307141.

281. Hoffmann B, Moebus S, Dragano N, et al. Residential traffic exposure and coronary heart disease: results from the Heinz Nixdorf Recall Study. Biomarkers. 2009;14:74–8. https://doi.org/10.1080/13547500902965096.

282. Bauer M, Moebus S, Mhlenkamp S, et al. Urban particulate matter air pollution is associated with subclinical atherosclerosis: results from the HNR (Heinz Nixdorf Recall) study. J Am Coll Cardiol. 2010;56:1803–8. https://doi.org/10.1016/j.jacc.2010.04.065.

283. Diez Roux AV, Auchincloss AH, Franklin TG, et al. Long-term exposure to ambient particulate matter and prevalence of subclinical atherosclerosis in the Multi-Ethnic Study of Atherosclerosis. Am J Epidemiol. 2008;167:667–75. https://doi.org/10.1093/aje/kwm359.

284. Hoffmann B, Moebus S, Mohlenkamp S, et al. Residential exposure to traffic is associated with coronary atherosclerosis. Circulation. 2007;116:489–96. https://doi.org/10.1161/CIRCULATIONAHA.107.693622.

285. Kalsch H, Hennig F, Moebus S, et al. Are air pollution and traffic noise independently associated with atherosclerosis: the Heinz Nixdorf Recall Study. Eur Heart J. 2014;35:853–60. https://doi.org/10.1093/eurheartj/eht426.

286. Künzli N, Jerrett M, Mack WJ, et al. Ambient air pollution and atherosclerosis in Los Angeles. Environ Health Perspect. 2005;113:201–6.

287. Künzli N, Jerrett M, Garcia-Esteban R, et al. Ambient air pollution and the progression of atherosclerosis in adults. PLoS One. 2010;5:e9096. https://doi.org/10.1371/journal.pone.0009096.

288. Rivera M, Basagaña X, Aguilera I, et al. Association between long-term exposure to traffic-related air pollution and subclinical atherosclerosis: the REGICOR study. Environ Health Perspect. 2013;121:223–30. https://doi.org/10.1289/ehp.1205146.

289. Wilker EH, Mittleman MA, Coull BA, et al. Long-term exposure to black carbon and carotid intima-media thickness: the normative aging study. Environ Health Perspect. 2013;121:1061–7. https://doi.org/10.1289/ehp.1104845.

290. Mustafic H, Jabre P, Caussin C, et al. Main air pollutants and myocardial infarction: a systematic review and meta-analysis. JAMA. 2012;307:713–21. https://doi.org/10.1001/jama.2012.126.

291. Nawrot TS, Perez L, Künzli N, et al. Public health importance of triggers of myocardial infarction: a comparative risk assessment. Lancet (London, England). 2011;377:732–40. https://doi.org/10.1016/S0140-6736(10)62296-9.

292. Clancy L, Goodman P, Sinclair H, Dockery DW. Effect of air-pollution control on death rates in Dublin, Ireland: an intervention study. Lancet. 2002;360:1210–4. https://doi.org/10.1016/S0140-6736(02)11281-5.

293. Bara C, Böthig D, Haverich A. Umweltmedizin: Feinstaubfolgen für das transplantierte Herz. Dtsch Arztebl. 2017;114:33. https://doi.org/10.3238/PersKardio.2017.03.31.07.

294. Li H, Chen R, Meng X, et al. Short-term exposure to ambient air pollution and coronary heart disease mortality in 8 Chinese cities. Int J Cardiol. 2015;197:265–70. https://doi.org/10.1016/j.ijcard.2015.06.050.

295. Wolf K, Schneider A, Breitner S, et al. Associations between short-term exposure to particulate matter and ultrafine particles and myocardial infarction in Augsburg, Germany. Int J Hyg Environ Health. 2015;218:535–42. https://doi.org/10.1016/j.ijheh.2015.05.002.

296. Powell H, Krall JR, Wang Y, et al. Ambient coarse particulate matter and hospital admissions in the medicare cohort air pollution study, 1999–2010. Environ Health Perspect. 2015;123:1152–8. https://doi.org/10.1289/ehp.1408720.

297. Faustini A, Alessandrini ER, Pey J, et al. Short-term effects of particulate matter on mortality during forest fires in Southern Europe: results of the MED-PARTICLES Project. Occup Environ Med. 2015;72:323–9. https://doi.org/10.1136/oemed-2014-102459.

298. Chang C-C, Chen P-S, Yang C-Y. Short-term effects of fine particulate air pollution on hospital admissions for cardiovascular diseases: a case-crossover study in a tropical city. J Toxicol Environ Heal Part A. 2015;78:267–77. https://doi.org/10.1080/15287394.2014.960044.

299. Talbott EO, Rager JR, Benson S, et al. A case-crossover analysis of the impact of PM2.5 on cardiovascular disease hospitalizations for selected CDC tracking states. Environ Res. 2014;134:455–65. https://doi.org/10.1016/j.envres.2014.06.018.

300. Pope CA, Muhlestein JB, May HT, et al. Ischemic heart disease events triggered by short-term exposure to fine particulate air pollution. Circulation. 2006;114:2443–8. https://doi.org/10.1161/CIRCULATIONAHA.106.636977.

301. Peters A, Dockery DW, Muller JE, Mittleman MA. Increased particulate air pollution and the triggering of myocardial infarction. Circulation. 2001;103:2810–5.

302. D'Ippoliti D, Forastiere F, Ancona C, et al. Air pollution and myocardial infarction in Rome. Epidemiology. 2003;14:528–35. https://doi.org/10.1097/01.ede.0000082046.22919.72.

303. Zanobetti A, Schwartz J. The effect of particulate air pollution on emergency admissions for myocardial infarction: a multicity case-crossover analysis. Environ Health Perspect. 2005;113:978–82.

304. von Klot S, Peters A, Aalto P, et al. Ambient air pollution is associated with increased risk of hospital cardiac readmissions of myocardial infarction survivors in five European cities. Circulation. 2005;112:3073–9. https://doi.org/10.1161/CIRCULATIONAHA.105.548743.

305. Vidale S, Arnaboldi M, Bosio V, et al. Short-term air pollution exposure and cardiovascular events: a 10-year study in the urban area of Como, Italy. Int J Cardiol. 2017;248:389–93. https://doi.org/10.1016/j.ijcard.2017.06.037.

306. Hart JE, Chiuve SE, Laden F, Albert CM. Roadway proximity and risk of sudden cardiac death in women. Circulation. 2014;130:1474–82. https://doi.org/10.1161/CIRCULATIONAHA.114.011489.

307. Kan H, London SJ, Chen G, et al. Season, sex, age, and education as modifiers of the effects of outdoor air pollution on daily mortality in Shanghai, China: the Public Health and Air Pollution in Asia (PAPA) study. Environ Health Perspect. 2008;116:1183–8. https://doi.org/10.1289/ehp.10851.

308. Hoffmann B, Weinmayr G, Hennig F, et al. Air quality, stroke, and coronary events: results of the Heinz Nixdorf Recall Study from the Ruhr Region. Dtsch Arztebl Int. 2015;112:195–201. https://doi.org/10.3238/arztebl.2015.0195.

309. Rosenbloom JI, Wilker EH, Mukamal KJ, et al. Residential proximity to major roadway and ten-year all-cause mortality after myocardial infarction. Circulation. 2012;125:2197–203. https://doi.org/10.1161/CIRCULATIONAHA.111.085811.

310. Miller MR, McLean SG, Duffin R, et al. Diesel exhaust particulate increases the size and complexity of lesions in atherosclerotic mice. Part Fibre Toxicol. 2013;10:61. https://doi.org/10.1186/1743-8977-10-61.

311. Bai N, Kido T, Suzuki H, et al. Changes in atherosclerotic plaques induced by inhalation of diesel exhaust. Atherosclerosis. 2011;216:299–306. https://doi.org/10.1016/j.atherosclerosis.2011.02.019.

312. Suwa T, Hogg JC, Quinlan KB, et al. Particulate air pollution induces progression of atherosclerosis. J Am Coll Cardiol. 2002;39:935–42.

313. Quan C, Sun Q, Lippmann M, Chen L-C. Comparative effects of inhaled diesel exhaust and ambient fine particles on inflammation, atherosclerosis, and vascular dysfunction. Inhal Toxicol. 2010;22:738–53. https://doi.org/10.3109/08958371003728057.

314. Sun Q, Wang A, Jin X, et al. Long-term air pollution exposure and acceleration of atherosclerosis and vascular inflammation in an animal model. JAMA. 2005;294:3003–10. https://doi.org/10.1001/jama.294.23.3003.

315. Brook RD, Brook JR, Urch B, et al. Inhalation of fine particulate air pollution and ozone causes acute arterial vasoconstriction in healthy adults. Circulation. 2002;105:1534–6.

316. Peretz A, Sullivan JH, Leotta DF, et al. Diesel exhaust inhalation elicits acute vasoconstriction in vivo. Environ Health Perspect. 2008;116:937–42. https://doi.org/10.1289/ehp.11027.

317. Lundbäck M, Mills NL, Lucking A, et al. Experimental exposure to diesel exhaust increases arterial stiffness in man. Part Fibre Toxicol. 2009;6:7. https://doi.org/10.1186/1743-8977-6-7.

318. Devlin RB, Ghio AJ, Kehrl H, et al. Elderly humans exposed to concentrated air pollution particles have decreased heart rate variability. Eur Respir J Suppl. 2003;40:76s–80s.

319. Gong H Jr, Linn WS, Sioutas C, et al. Controlled exposures of healthy and asthmatic volunteers to concentrated ambient fine particles in Los Angeles. Inhal Toxicol. 2003;15:305–25. https://doi.org/10.1080/08958370304455.

320. Gong H, Linn WS, Terrell SL, et al. Altered heart-rate variability in asthmatic and healthy volunteers exposed to concentrated ambient coarse particles. Inhal Toxicol. 2004;16:335–43. https://doi.org/10.1080/08958370490439470.

321. Gong H, Linn WS, Clark KW, et al. Exposures of healthy and asthmatic volunteers to concentrated ambient ultrafine particles in Los Angeles. Inhal Toxicol. 2008;20:533–45. https://doi.org/10.1080/08958370801911340.

322. Brook RD, Shin HH, Bard RL, et al. Exploration of the rapid effects of personal fine particulate matter exposure on arterial hemodynamics and vascular function during the same day. Environ Health Perspect. 2011;119:688–94.

323. Urch B, Silverman F, Corey P, et al. Acute blood pressure responses in healthy adults during controlled air pollution exposures. Environ Health Perspect. 2005;113:1052–5.

324. Mills NL, Törnqvist H, Gonzalez MC, et al. Ischemic and thrombotic effects of dilute diesel-exhaust inhalation in men with coronary heart disease. N Engl J Med. 2007;357:1075–82. https://doi.org/10.1056/NEJMoa066314.

325. Törnqvist H, Mills NL, Gonzalez M, et al. Persistent endothelial dysfunction in humans after diesel exhaust inhalation. Am J Respir Crit Care Med. 2007;176:395–400. https://doi.org/10.1164/rccm.200606-872OC.

326. Lucking AJ, Lundback M, Mills NL, et al. Diesel exhaust inhalation increases thrombus formation in man. Eur Heart J. 2008;29:3043–51. https://doi.org/10.1093/eurheartj/ehn464.

327. Li H, Cai J, Chen R, et al. Particulate matter exposure and stress hormone levels: a randomized, double-blind, crossover trial of air purification. Circulation. 2017;136:618–27. https://doi.org/10.1161/CIRCULATIONAHA.116.026796.

328. Wang Z, Klipfell E, Bennett BJ, et al. Gut flora metabolism of phosphatidylcholine promotes cardiovascular disease. Nature. 2011;472:57–63. https://doi.org/10.1038/nature09922.

329. Wang Z, Roberts AB, Buffa JA, et al. Non-lethal inhibition of gut microbial trimethylamine production for the treatment of atherosclerosis. Cell. 2015;163:1585–95. https://doi.org/10.1016/j.cell.2015.11.055.

330. Tang WHW, Hazen SL. The contributory role of gut microbiota in cardiovascular disease. J Clin Invest. 2014;124:4204–11. https://doi.org/10.1172/JCI72331.

331. Koeth RA, Wang Z, Levison BS, et al. Intestinal microbiota metabolism of L-carnitine, a nutrient in red meat, promotes atherosclerosis. Nat Med. 2013;19:576–85. https://doi.org/10.1038/nm.3145.

332. Tang WHW, Wang Z, Levison BS, et al. Intestinal microbial metabolism of phosphatidylcholine and cardiovascular risk. N Engl J Med. 2013;368:1575–84. https://doi.org/10.1056/NEJMoa1109400.

333. Zhu W, Gregory JC, Org E, et al. Gut microbial metabolite TMAO enhances platelet hyperreactivity and thrombosis risk. Cell. 2016;165:111–24. https://doi.org/10.1016/j.cell.2016.02.011.

334. Al-Waiz M, Mikov M, Mitchell SC, Smith RL. The exogenous origin of trimethylamine in the mouse. Metabolism. 1992;41:135–6. https://doi.org/10.1016/0026-0495(92)90140-6.

335. Gregory JC, Buffa JA, Org E, et al. Transmission of atherosclerosis susceptibility with gut microbial transplantation. J Biol Chem. 2015;290:5647–60. https://doi.org/10.1074/jbc.M114.618249.

336. Jaiswal S, Natarajan P, Silver AJ, et al. Clonal hematopoiesis and risk of atherosclerotic cardiovascular disease. N Engl J Med. 2017. https://doi.org/10.1056/NEJMoa1701719.

337. Jaiswal S, Fontanillas P, Flannick J, et al. Age-related clonal hematopoiesis associated with adverse outcomes. N Engl J Med. 2014;371:2488–98. https://doi.org/10.1056/NEJMoa1408617.

338. Steensma DP, Bejar R, Jaiswal S, et al. Clonal hematopoiesis of indeterminate potential and its distinction from myelodysplastic syndromes. Blood. 2015;126:9–16. https://doi.org/10.1182/blood-2015-03-631747.

339. Acuna-Hidalgo R, Sengul H, Steehouwer M, et al. Ultra-sensitive sequencing identifies high prevalence of clonal hematopoiesis-associated mutations throughout adult life. Am J Hum Genet. 2017;101:50–64. https://doi.org/10.1016/j.ajhg.2017.05.013.

340. Fuster JJ, MacLauchlan S, Zuriaga MA, et al. Clonal hematopoiesis associated with TET2 deficiency accelerates atherosclerosis development in mice. Science. 2017;355:842–847. https://doi.org/10.1126/science.aag1381.

341. Virchow R. Cellular pathology; 1860.

342. Libby P, Okamoto Y, Rocha VZ, Folco E. Inflammation in atherosclerosis. Circ J. 2010;74:213–20. https://doi.org/10.1253/circj.CJ-09-0706.

343. Munro JM, Cotran RS. The pathogenesis of atherosclerosis: atherogenesis and inflammation. Lab Invest. 1988;58:249–61.

344. Emerging Risk Factors Collaboration, Kaptoge S, Di Angelantonio E, et al. C-reactive protein concentration and risk of coronary heart disease, stroke, and mortality: an individual participant meta-analysis. Lancet (London, England). 2010;375:132–40. https://doi.org/10.1016/S0140-6736(09)61717-7.

345. Emerging Risk Factors Collaboration, Kaptoge S, Di Angelantonio E, et al. C-reactive protein, fibrinogen, and cardiovascular disease prediction. N Engl J Med. 2012;367:1310–20. https://doi.org/10.1056/NEJMoa1107477.

346. Wennberg P, Wensley F, Di Angelantonio E, et al. Haemostatic and inflammatory markers are independently associated with myocardial infarction in men and women. Thromb Res. 2012;129:68–73. https://doi.org/10.1016/j.thromres.2011.05.015.

347. Ridker PM, Hennekens CH, Buring JE, Rifai N. C-reactive protein and other markers of inflammation in the prediction of cardiovascular disease in women. N Engl J Med. 2000;342:836–43. https://doi.org/10.1056/NEJM200003233421202.
348. Koenig W, Sund M, Fröhlich M, et al. C-reactive protein, a sensitive marker of inflammation, predicts future risk of coronary heart disease in initially healthy middle-aged men: results from the MONICA (Monitoring Trends and Determinants in Cardiovascular Disease) Augsburg Cohort Study, 1984 to 1992. Circulation. 1999;99:237–42.
349. Kuller LH, Tracy RP, Shaten J, Meilahn EN. Relation of C-reactive protein and coronary heart disease in the MRFIT nested case-control study. Multiple risk factor intervention trial. Am J Epidemiol. 1996;144:537–47.
350. C-Reactive Protein Coronary Heart Disease Genetics Collaboration, Wensley F, Gao P, et al. Association between C reactive protein and coronary heart disease: mendelian randomisation analysis based on individual participant data. BMJ. 2011;342:d548. https://doi.org/10.1136/bmj.d548.
351. Sheedy FJ, Grebe A, Rayner KJ, et al. CD36 coordinates NLRP3 inflammasome activation by facilitating intracellular nucleation of soluble ligands into particulate ligands in sterile inflammation. Nat Immunol. 2013;14:812–20. https://doi.org/10.1038/ni.2639.
352. Hoseini Z, Sepahvand F, Rashidi B, et al. NLRP3 inflammasome: its regulation and involvement in atherosclerosis. J Cell Physiol. 2017. https://doi.org/10.1002/jcp.25930.
353. Després JP. Health consequences of visceral obesity. Ann Med. 2001;33:534–41.
354. Savoia C, Schiffrin EL. Inflammation in hypertension. Curr Opin Intern Med. 2006;5:245–51. https://doi.org/10.1097/01.mnh.0000203189.57513.76.
355. Altman R. Risk factors in coronary atherosclerosis athero-inflammation: the meeting point. Thromb J. 2003;1:1–11. https://doi.org/10.1186/1477-9560-1-4.
356. Donath MY, Shoelson SE. Type 2 diabetes as an inflammatory disease. Nat Rev Immunol. 2011;11:98–107. https://doi.org/10.1038/nri2925.
357. Silverstein DM. Inflammation in chronic kidney disease: role in the progression of renal and cardiovascular disease. Pediatr Nephrol. 2009;24:1445–52. https://doi.org/10.1007/s00467-008-1046-0.
358. Lee J, Taneja V, Vassallo R. Cigarette smoking and inflammation: cellular and molecular mechanisms. J Dent Res. 2012;91:142–9. https://doi.org/10.1177/0022034511421200.
359. Bohula EA, Giugliano RP, Cannon CP, et al. Achievement of dual low-density lipoprotein cholesterol and high-sensitivity c-reactive protein targets more frequent with the addition of ezetimibe to simvastatin and associated with better outcomes in IMPROVE-IT. Circulation. 2015;132:1224–33. https://doi.org/10.1161/CIRCULATIONAHA.115.018381.
360. Scirica BM, Cannon CP, Sabatine MS, et al. Concentrations of C-reactive protein and B-type natriuretic peptide 30 days after acute coronary syndromes independently predict hospitalization for heart failure and cardiovascular death. Clin Chem. 2009;55:265–73. https://doi.org/10.1373/clinchem.2008.117192.
361. Ridker PM, Danielson E, Fonseca FAH, et al. Rosuvastatin to prevent vascular events in men and women with elevated C-reactive protein. N Engl J Med. 2008;359:2195–207. https://doi.org/10.1056/NEJMoa0807646.
362. Shishehbor MH, Hazen SL. JUPITER to earth: a statin helps people with normal LDL-C and high hs-CRP, but what does it mean? Cleve Clin J Med. 2009;76:37–44. https://doi.org/10.3949/ccjm.75a.08105.
363. Ridker PM, Thuren T, Zalewski A, Libby P. Interleukin-1β inhibition and the prevention of recurrent cardiovascular events: rationale and design of the Canakinumab Antiinflammatory Thrombosis Outcomes Study (CANTOS). Am Heart J. 2011;162:597–605. https://doi.org/10.1016/j.ahj.2011.06.012.
364. Ridker PM, Everett BM, Thuren T, et al. Antiinflammatory therapy with canakinumab for atherosclerotic disease. N Engl J Med. 2017;377:1119–31. https://doi.org/10.1056/NEJMoa1707914.

365. Hansson GK. Inflammation and atherosclerosis-The end of a controversy. Circulation. 2017. https://doi.org/10.1161/CIRCULATIONAHA.117.030484.
366. Baylis RA, Gomez D, Mallat Z, et al. The CANTOS trial one important step for clinical cardiology but a giant leap for vascular biology. Arterioscler Thromb Vasc Biol. 2017;37:e174–7. https://doi.org/10.1161/ATVBAHA.117.310097.
367. Baber U, Mehran R, Sartori S, et al. Prevalence, impact, and predictive value of detecting subclinical coronary and carotid atherosclerosis in asymptomatic adults: the bioimage study. J Am Coll Cardiol. 2015;65:1065–74. https://doi.org/10.1016/j.jacc.2015.01.017.
368. Wilkins JT, Ning H, Berry J, et al. Lifetime risk and years lived free of total cardiovascular disease. JAMA. 2012;308:1795. https://doi.org/10.1001/jama.2012.14312.
369. Rothman KJ, Greenland S. Causation and causal inference in epidemiology. Am J Public Health. 2005;95:S144–50. https://doi.org/10.2105/AJPH.2004.059204.

Chapter 3
The Effect of Growth and Aging on the Vascular Architecture

3.1 The Blood Vasculature

Blood vessel walls are composed of three layers: the intima, the media, and the adventitia. The vascular architecture changes with growth and aging [1]. At birth, the innermost intima in humans is comprised solely of a single endothelial layer attached to an underlying matrix surrounded by an internal elastic lamina [2]. The media has circularly arranged lamellar units consisting of smooth muscle cells, connective tissue, and elastic fibers. The outer adventitia is composed of collagen-rich connective tissue containing fibroblasts, perivascular nerves, pericytes, adipocytes, as well as resident populations of macrophages, T-cells, B-cells, mast cells, and dendritic cells that carry out important surveillance and innate immune functions [3, 4]. Separating the intima from the media and the media from the adventitia are elastic membranes. In the past decade or so, it was discovered that the intima, media, and adventitia contain vascular wall-resident stem cells capable of differentiating into both vascular and nonvascular (e.g., macrophages, follicular dendritic cells) cell types [5].

When blood vessels do not exceed a critical wall thickness, luminal oxygen and nutrients enter the vessel wall aided by a permeable endothelial layer and high intra-arterial pressure. Since under physiological conditions the blood pressure in the main arterial lumen is higher than the pressure in the surrounding tissue, the blood solutes tend to diffuse from the main lumen to the adventitia [6]. This process is defined by Darcy's Law, which describes diffusion of a solute through a porous medium when subjected to a pressure gradient [6, 7]. Certain biomechanical factors can trigger vascular growth. For instance, wall tension (W) is determined by vessel diameter (r), blood pressure (p), and vessel wall thickness (t).

$$W = (rp)/t \qquad (3.1)$$

© Springer Nature Switzerland AG 2019
A. Haverich and E. C. Boyle, *Atherosclerosis Pathogenesis and Microvascular Dysfunction*, https://doi.org/10.1007/978-3-030-20245-3_3

Accordingly, wall tension increases along with blood pressure and vessel radius, resulting in an increase in wall thickness. This implies that large arteries must have thicker walls than small arteries in order to withstand the level of tension. Mechanosensors detect these hemodynamic forces and transmit them to biochemical signals that result in endothelial and smooth muscle cell proliferation. From very early experiments in dogs, where a longitudinal incision was performed in the adventitial layer, we know that this tunica is primarily responsible for the mechanical stability of the arterial wall [8]. This finding, often observed in surgery for aortic dissection, also elucidates the critical role of the adventitial layer in arterial aneurysm formation.

Richard Thoma was the first to report that the intima of the aorta and coronary arteries increased in thickness according to growth and age [9]. Owing to the diligent and detailed work of Kapitoline Wolkoff, we now know the normal postnatal development of the human coronary artery from birth to its normal adult architecture [1]. Similar to growth rings of a tree, **with age, the number of intimal cell layers increases, starting with 1–2 cell layers at birth, 10–15 layers by age 15, and 25–30 layers by age 25–30.** The process of increasing cell layers is called diffuse intimal thickening (DIT) or intimal hyperplasia (Fig. 3.1). Wolkoff also observed DIT in various animals and noticed the extent of DIT seemed to correlate

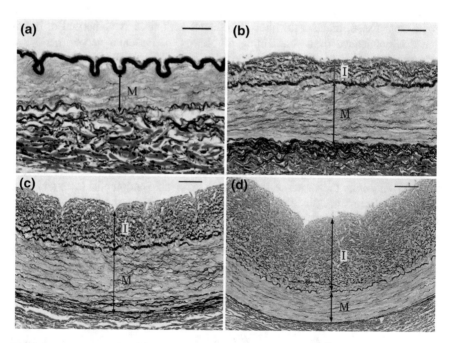

Fig. 3.1 Age-related diffuse intimal thickening in the proximal coronary artery of humans. **a** 7-day old's right coronary artery, **b** 5-year old's left anterior descending artery (LAD), **c** 15-year old's LAD, and **d** 29-year old's LAD. Scale bars in **a**, **b**, **c**, and **d** represent 25, 50, 50, and 100 μm, respectively. I, intima; M, media. Reproduced from [12]

with both age and body size. She noted that the age-related increase in DIT could be put in the following order: mice, rats, rabbits, cats, dogs, monkeys, cows, and horses [10]. Wolkoff's mentor, Anitschow, the Russian pathologist famous for his work on cholesterol and atherosclerosis praised her study and reemphasized her conclusions in his book chapter *Arteriosclerosis: A Survey of the Problem* [11]:

"...it is important to remember that thickening of the intima also occurs in experimental animals as a purely physiological phenomena in the process of aging."

Despite these early indications that DIT was part of normal development, and found in humans and animals alike, it was later mistakenly associated with early disease development. It has been suggested that the reason for this association resulted from differences in tissue sampling and preparation [13]. Improperly fixed vessels were interpreted as stenosed or occluded because the intima protruded into the lumen as a result of the vessel's collapsed and contracted state. Stary et al. also pointed out that thickening at specific sites can be an adaptation to reduced shear stress. Importantly, adaptive intimal thickening occurs regardless of whether high concentrations of cholesterol are present or not. Today, DIT is understood to be a normal developmental process universally associated with artery growth [13]. Nevertheless, in heart disease staging, human lesions are considered to originate from preexisting intimal thickening [14]. Therefore, the idea that DIT is in some way pathological perseveres.

3.2 The Blood Microvasculature

Nutrition of thin-walled blood vessels occurs through diffusion alone. However, at a critical thickness of 29 lamellar units in the media or greater than a diameter of 0.5 mm, diffusion from the lumen becomes insufficient [15, 16].

"When the intima of the coronary artery exceeds a certain thickness parts must either die or develop secondary blood supply." (Geoffrey R. Osborn, 1963) [17]

Upon exceeding this critical dimension, it is believed that hypoxic conditions in the outer media and adventitia initiate angiogenic processes and vasa vasorum formation when this critical thickness is exceeded [2]. The name "vasa vasorum" is derived from Latin, meaning "the vessels of the vessels". They are blood microvessels that supply the walls of medium and large arteries and veins with nutrients and oxygen [18]. In addition, they participate in removing systemic waste products [19]. Vasa vasorum first appear confined to the adventitia in young subjects. With advancing age and increasing wall thickness, they enter into the outer two-thirds of the media [20–22]. Therefore, vasa vasorum penetrate and nourish the adventitia and outer media, while the luminal blood supplies nourishment to the inner 0.5 mm [23–25] (Fig. 3.2).

There are three different types of vasa vasorum [26]. The most common (96%) are vasa vasorum externae, which originate from larger branches of the parent

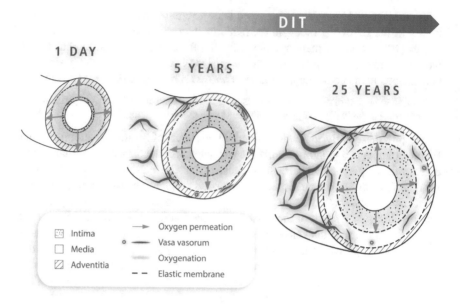

Fig. 3.2 Growth-dependent development of vasa vasorum facilitates nourishment and oxygenation of the vessel wall layers. DIT, diffuse intimal thickening

vessels. For example, vasa vasorum in the ascending aorta can originate from the brachiocephalic and coronary arteries, the intercostal branches in the descending thoracic artery, the lumbar and mesenteric arteries in the abdominal aorta, or from the bifurcation segments of epicardial vessels in coronary arteries [20]. There are also venous vasa vasorum that drain the arterial wall into veins, and the very rare vasa vasorum internae that originate from the main lumen of the parent artery [24, 25, 27, 28]. Vasa vasorum are further categorized into first- and second-order microvessels. First-order vasa vasorum run longitudinally parallel to the vessel while second-order microvessels are associated with neovascularization and branch from first-order vasa within the vessel wall [27–29].

The normal size of human vasa vasorum varies between 80 and 150 μm, and their plasticity is extremely high. Through microembolism experiments of normal porcine coronary arteries, Gössl et al. elegantly showed that **vasa vasorum do not form a plexus, but are rather functional end arteries** [30]. By definition, these are not linked to other vessels' perfusion territories and thus vasa vasorum supply nutrients and oxygen to a confined subintimal area. Vasa vasorum can be transiently compressed by the surrounding arterial wall. In addition, they regulate their own tone and vascular perfusion because they are surrounded by their own vascular smooth muscle cells and connective tissue [6, 19, 23, 31, 32].

The amount of vasa vasorum is adaptive to the oxygen concentrations in the vessel wall. As mentioned, this can be influenced by thickness of the vessel wall but is also determined by luminal oxygen concentrations. For instance, veins possess far more vasa vasorum than arteries as they must compensate for the fact that veins are carrying blood that is low in oxygen. Even more striking are the examples of children with congenital heart disease (e.g., cyanotic blue babies) which display a significant amount of vasa vasorum in the ascending thoracic aorta, where there are normally none in healthy children of the same age.

3.3 The Lymphatic Vasculature

Running almost parallel with the blood's circulation is the lymphatic system. Lymphatics consist of a network of initial lymphatics that drain into pre-collecting and subsequently collecting lymphatic vessels [33]. The initial lymphatics consist solely of an endothelium anchored to an underlying basement membrane via collagen fibers. Fluid enters into these blind-ended capillaries by absorption aided by relatively permeable endothelial junctions [34] and a pressure gradient that favors fluid movement from the interstitium into the lymphatics. The smallest pre-collectors have sparse smooth muscle coverage and contain valves that maintain unidirectional flow of lymph into the contractile collecting lymphatic vessels. There fluid is propelled by the muscular action of skeletal muscles, respiration, and the smooth muscles of the larger collecting lymphatic vessels themselves. The vessel wall of the collecting vessels is thin, but divided into recognizable intimal, medial, and adventitial layers. Collecting lymphatics then pump the lymph to regional lymph nodes and on to the thoracic or right lymphatic duct where fluid re-enters the blood circulation.

One of the lymphatic system's most important roles is tissue fluid homeostasis in that it transports excess interstitial fluid back into the blood circulation. Lymphatics also take part in lipid absorption and lipid metabolism and are involved in immune surveillance by transporting immune cells and antigens to regional lymph nodes. Similar to vasa vasorum, lymphatic microvessels are present in the adventitia of larger blood vessels, with densities proportional to intimal thickness [35–37]. The intramural arterial and perivascular lymphatic beds have other critical functions including reverse cholesterol transport (RCT) out of the artery wall [38]. Excess cellular cholesterol in the interstitial space is attached to HDL and transported via the lymph to the bloodstream and back to the liver to ultimately be excreted [39].

Interestingly and often overlooked is the fact that larger lymphatic vessel walls also have their own blood supply in the form of vasa vasorum [40–42]. Similar to blood vessel vasa vasorum, lymphatic vessel vasa vasorum lie in the adventitia (Fig. 3.3). The size of lymphatic vessels that possess these microvessels is much smaller than that of a corresponding blood vessel wall [42], which could be related to the lower oxygen tension in lymphatic vessels compared to arteries. Vasa vasorum observed in lymphatic vessels have diameters as small as 0.1 mm.

"Lymphatic vessels possess a special blood-supply when possessing a caliber far below that of blood-vessels which have vasa vasorum." [43]

Fig. 3.3 Scanning electron microscopy showing that the thoracic duct is richly supplied with blood microvessels. Pictured is the abluminal side of the adventitia of a human thoracic duct. Arterial vasa vasorum (*red*), venous vasa vasorum (*blue*), and capillaries (*yellow*) are distributed within this lymphatic vessel. Reproduced from [43]

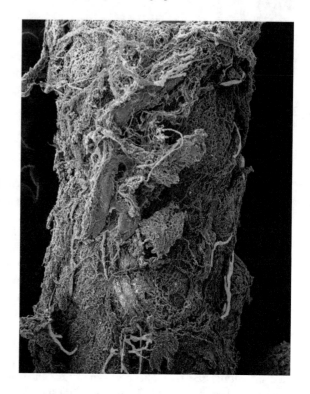

Now that we have a handle on the architecture of the blood and lymphatic vasculature during health, we will turn our attention in the next chapter to what happens during atherosclerotic disease. **The microvasculature that lies in both blood and lymphatic vessels is a neglected area of research** and an often ignored aspect of the pathophysiology of cardiovascular disease. In the case of atherosclerosis, the primary focus is always on the endothelium of the parent vessel when, as we will suggest, it is the endothelium of the vasa vasorum that is more susceptible to dysfunction during all stages of disease (initiation, progression, and rupture).

References

1. Wolkoff K. Ueber die histologische Struktur der Coronararterien des menschlichen Herzens. Virchows Arch. 1923;241:42–58.
2. Boyle EC, Sedding DG, Haverich A. Targeting vasa vasorum dysfunction to prevent atherosclerosis. Vascul Pharmacol. 2017;96–98:5–10. https://doi.org/10.1016/j.vph.2017.08.003.
3. Majesky MW, Dong XR, Hoglund V, et al. The adventitia: a dynamic interface containing resident progenitor cells. Arterioscler Thromb Vasc Biol. 2011;31:1530–9. https://doi.org/10.1161/ATVBAHA.110.221549.
4. Galkina E, Kadl A, Sanders J, et al. Lymphocyte recruitment into the aortic wall before and during development of atherosclerosis is partially L-selectin dependent. J Exp Med. 2006;203:1273–82. https://doi.org/10.1084/jem.20052205.

5. Wörsdörfer P, Mekala SR, Bauer J, et al. The vascular adventitia: an endogenous, omnipresent source of stem cells in the body. Pharmacol Ther. 2017;171:13–29. https://doi.org/10.1016/j.pharmthera.2016.07.017.

6. Ritman E, Lerman A. The dynamic vasa vasorum. Cardiovasc Res. 2007;75:649–58. https://doi.org/10.1016/j.cardiores.2007.06.020.

7. Bear J. Dynamics of Fluids in Porous Media; 1972.

8. Winternitz MC, Thomas RMM, LeCompte P. The biology of arteriosclerosis. Springfield, IL: Charles C Thomas; 1938.

9. Thoma R. Über die Abhängigkeit der Bindegewebsneubildung in der Arterienintima von den mechanischen Bedingungen des Blutumlaufs. Virchows Arch. 1883;93:443–505.

10. Wolkoff K. Ueber die Altersveraenderungen der Arterien bei Tieren. Virchows. 1924;252:208–28.

11. Anitschow NN. Experimental arteriosclerosis in animals. In: Crowdy EV, editor. Arteriosclerosis: a survey of the problem. New York: MacMillan Publishing; 1933. p. 271–322.

12. Nakashima Y, Chen Y-X, Kinukawa N, Sueishi K. Distributions of diffuse intimal thickening in human arteries: preferential expression in atherosclerosis-prone arteries from an early age. Virchows Arch. 2002;441:279–88. https://doi.org/10.1007/s00428-002-0605-1.

13. Stary HC, Blankenhorn DH, Chandler AB, et al. A definition of the intima of human arteries and of its atherosclerosis- prone regions. A report from the Committee on Vascular Lesions of the Council on Arteriosclerosis, American Heart Association. Arterioscler Thromb Vasc Biol. 1992;12:120–34. https://doi.org/10.1161/01.ATV.12.1.120.

14. Virmani R, Kolodgie FD, Burke AP, et al. Lessons from sudden coronary death: a comprehensive morphological classification scheme for atherosclerotic lesions. Arterioscler Thromb Vasc Biol. 2000;20:1262–75.

15. Geiringer E. Intimal vascularisation and artherosclerosis. J Pathol Bacteriol. 1951;63:201–11. https://doi.org/10.1002/path.1700630204.

16. Wolinsky H, Glagov S. Comparison of abdominal and thoracic aortic medial structure in mammals. Circ Res. 1969;25:677–86. https://doi.org/10.1161/01.RES.25.6.677.

17. Osborn GR. The incubation period of coronary thrombosis. London: Butterworths; 1963.

18. Martin H. Considérations générales sur la pathogénie des scléroses dystrophiques. Revue de Medecine. 1886;1–26.

19. Xu J, Lu X, Shi G-P. Vasa vasorum in atherosclerosis and clinical significance. Int J Mol Sci. 2015;16:11574–608. https://doi.org/10.3390/ijms160511574.

20. Clarke JA. An x-ray microscopic study of the postnatal development of the vasa vasorum in the human aorta. J Anat. 1965;99:877–89.

21. Clarke JA. An x-ray microscopic study of the blood-supply to the aortic bifurcation and common iliac arteries. Br J Surg. 1966;53:354–8.

22. Wolinsky H, Glagov S. Nature of species differences in the medial distribution of aortic vasa vasorum in mammals. Circ Res. 1967;20:409–21. https://doi.org/10.1161/01.RES.20.4.409.

23. Heistad DD, Marcus ML, Law EG, et al. Regulation of blood flow to the aortic media in dogs. J Clin Invest. 1978;62:133–40. https://doi.org/10.1172/JCI109097.

24. Heistad DD, Marcus ML. Role of vasa vasorum in nourishment of the aorta. J Vasc Res. 1979;16:225–38. https://doi.org/10.1159/000158209.

25. Heistad DD, Marcus ML, Larsen GE, Armstrong ML. Role of vasa vasorum in nourishment of the aortic wall. Am J Physiol. 1981;240:H781–7.

26. Schoenberger F, Mueller A. On the vascularization of the bovine aortic wall. Helv Physiol Pharmacol Acta. 1960;18:136–50.

27. Kwon HM, Sangiorgi G, Ritman EL, et al. Adventitial vasa vasorum in balloon-injured coronary arteries: visualization and quantitation by a microscopic three-dimensional computed tomography technique. J Am Coll Cardiol. 1998;32:2072–9. https://doi.org/10.1016/S0735-1097(98)00482-3.

28. Gössl M, Rosol M, Malyar NM, et al. Functional anatomy and hemodynamic characteristics of vasa vasorum in the walls of porcine coronary arteries. Anat Rec Part A Discov Mol Cell Evol Biol. 2003;272A:526–37. https://doi.org/10.1002/ar.a.10060.

29. Mulligan-Kehoe MJ. The vasa vasorum in diseased and nondiseased arteries. AJP Hear Circ Physiol. 2010;298:H295–305. https://doi.org/10.1152/ajpheart.00884.2009.

30. Gössl M, Malyar NM, Rosol M, et al. Impact of coronary vasa vasorum functional structure on coronary vessel wall perfusion distribution. Am J Physiol Hear Circ Physiol. 2003;285:H2019–26. https://doi.org/10.1152/ajpheart.00399.2003.

31. Scotland R, Vallance P, Ahluwalia A. Endothelin alters the reactivity of vasa vasorum: mechanisms and implications for conduit vessel physiology and pathophysiology. Br J Pharmacol. 1999;128:1229–34. https://doi.org/10.1038/sj.bjp.0702930.

32. Scotland R, Vallance P, Ahluwalia A. On the regulation of tone in vasa vasorum. Cardiovasc Res. 1999;41:237–45.

33. Adamczyk LA, Gordon K, Kholová I, et al. Lymph vessels: the forgotten second circulation in health and disease. Virchows Arch. 2016;469:3–17.

34. Baluk P, Fuxe J, Hashizume H, et al. Functionally specialized junctions between endothelial cells of lymphatic vessels. J Exp Med. 2007;204:2349–62. https://doi.org/10.1084/jem.20062596.

35. Drozdz K, Janczak D, Dziegiel P, et al. Adventitial lymphatics of internal carotid artery in healthy and atherosclerotic vessels. Folia Histochem Cytobiol. 2008;46:433–6. https://doi.org/10.2478/v10042-008-0083-7.

36. Drozdz K, Janczak D, Dziegiel P, et al. Adventitial lymphatics and atherosclerosis. Lymphology. 2012;45:26–33.

37. Sano M, Unno N, Sasaki T, et al. Topologic distributions of vasa vasorum and lymphatic vasa vasorum in the aortic adventitia–implications for the prevalence of aortic diseases. Atherosclerosis. 2016;247:127–34. https://doi.org/10.1016/j.atherosclerosis.2016.02.007.

38. Huang L-H, Elvington A, Randolph GJ. The role of the lymphatic system in cholesterol transport. Front Pharmacol. 2015;6:182. https://doi.org/10.3389/fphar.2015.00182.

39. Martel C, Li W, Fulp B, et al. Lymphatic vasculature mediates macrophage reverse cholesterol transport in mice. J Clin Invest. 2013;123:1571–9. https://doi.org/10.1172/JCI63685.

40. Dogiel A. Über ein die Lymphgefäße umspinnendes Netz von Blutkapillaren. Arch für Mikroskopische Anat. 1879;17:334.

41. Dogiel A. Über die Beziehungen zwischen Blut- und Lymphgefäßen. Arch f Mik Anat. 1883;22:608.

42. Evans HM. The blood supply of lymphatic vessels in man. Am J Anat. 1907;7:195–208.

43. Chiba T, Narita H, Shimoda H. Fine structure of human thoracic duct as revealed by light and scanning electron microscopy. Biomed Res. 2017;38:197–205. https://doi.org/10.2220/biomedres.38.197.

Chapter 4
Incriminating Evidence for the Role of the Microvasculature in Atherosclerosis

4.1 General

The dogma of atherosclerosis development can be divided into four steps: (i) endothelial dysfunction due to factors such as inflammation and high levels of serum LDL, (ii) deposition of lipids from the luminal blood into the arterial intima resulting in fatty streak formation, (iii) migration of leukocytes and smooth muscle cells into the vessel wall, and (iv) foam cell formation and the degradation of extracellular matrix [1]. During the progression of a plaque, endothelial cells, macrophages, and smooth muscle cells die, leading to the formation of a lipid-rich necrotic core covered by a fibrous cap. In later stages of plaque progression, many plaques become calcified while plaque destabilization and rupture result in the clinical complications associated with atherosclerosis. A growing body of evidence suggests that the microvasculature plays a central role in the pathogenesis of atherosclerosis. In this chapter, we will discuss both vasa vasorum and lymphatic microvasculature dysfunction during disease progression. And while the most research focuses on the endothelium of the parent vessel, we make a case that it is the endothelium of the vasa vasorum that is more susceptible to dysfunction during all stages of disease.

4.2 Vasa Vasorum: At the Right Place at the Right Time

Different vascular beds show a different susceptibility to atherosclerosis. The aorta and proximal coronary arteries are the most frequently affected sites, with the carotid and femoral arteries also often being affected. Interestingly, certain arterial segments are almost always spared from disease. This fact allows these segments to be used as bypass material (e.g., internal thoracic artery, radial artery).

© Springer Nature Switzerland AG 2019
A. Haverich and E. C. Boyle, *Atherosclerosis Pathogenesis and Microvascular Dysfunction*, https://doi.org/10.1007/978-3-030-20245-3_4

Even within diseased vessels themselves, plaques display a distinct localization in that adventitial conditions, such as the intramuscular course of a coronary artery (i.e., intramyocardial bridge) results in segmental protection from disease. Bypass grafting clearly demonstrates the impact of the type and location of a vessel. Radial arteries are rarely prone to atherosclerosis in situ, but can develop atherosclerosis when used in bypass surgery [2], while this almost never occurs when internal thoracic arteries are used [3]. The early failure rate of internal thoracic artery grafts is only 0.7% compared to 5.3% for radial arteries [2]. This difference could be the result of distinct mechanical properties of each artery or the fact that the adventitia of internal thoracic arteries has few vasa vasorum.

Vasa vasorum are distinctly distributed in the arterial system, with far less decoration of distal, smaller arteries compared to larger arteries closer to the heart [4–9]. Using optical coherence tomography, Nishimiya and colleagues found no adventitial vasa vasorum at the myocardial bridge in the left anterior descending arteries while they were present in the proximal and distal reference segments (Fig. 4.1) [10]. In pigs, Galili et al. showed that the vasa vasorum density was highest in coronary arteries, intermediate in renal arteries and carotid arteries, and lowest in femoral arteries [5]. A similar pattern was also observed for the ratio of second- to first-order vasa vasorum. There is abundant evidence that the prevalence and severity of atherosclerotic lesions correlate with the location and density of vasa vasorum [4, 5, 9, 11–14]. In ApoE-deficient mice, Langheinrich et al. demonstrated that lesion volume was associated with adventitial vasa vasorum neovascularization and that the site of atherosclerosis was connected to the appearance of vasa vasorum [11, 12]. Site-specific differences were observed in density and size, with vasa vasorum developing along the aorta proceeding distally from the ascending aorta and aortic arch [9]. Conversely, areas normally spared from atherosclerosis like the internal thoracic artery, radial artery, and intramyocardial bridge conspicuously lack vasa vasorum [5, 10, 15]. Hence, we propose that the

Fig. 4.1 Three-dimensional optical coherence tomography showing the absence of vasa vasorum at the myocardial bridge despite abundant adventitial vasa vasorum both proximal and distal to this segment. VV, vasa vasorum; MB, myocardial bridge. Reproduced from [10]

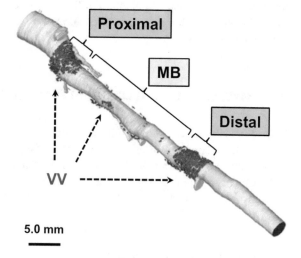

differential distribution of vasa vasorum likely plays an important role in the site specificity of disease manifestation.

It was previously thought that due to Lame's Law, blood flow from vasa vasorum deeper than the outer two-thirds of the media was not possible because of the compressive force within the arterial wall [16]. However, in atherogenic plaques, neovessels extend into the inner media and intima [17–20]. The predominant dogma in the field believes that lipids enter the intimal layer through damage to the parental vessel endothelium. If this were the case, deposition of lipids should initially be seen adjacent to the arterial lumen and in all arteries, large and small without site specificity. However, the elegant studies of Nakashima and colleagues demonstrate that **during very early plaque development, lipids are exclusively deposited in the deeper layers of the intima away from the endothelium** (Fig. 4.2) [21]. These intriguing observations counter the widely held belief that cholesterol enters the vessel wall via the endothelium of the parent vessel and rather supports the outside-in development of plaque formation [22]. **Due to their anatomical position, vasa vasorum are perfectly situated to be involved in delivering pro-atherosclerotic components into the deeper layers of the intima during early stages of disease** [23].

And while the initial presence of vasa vasorum is not itself pathological, but is rather a normal physiological response triggered by the oxygenation and nutritional needs of the larger vessel, there is increasing evidence to support the idea that vasa vasorum dysfunction is a key mediator of atherosclerosis initiation. Supporting this hypothesis, many studies have shown that the inappropriate growth, focal expansion, and appearance of larger convoluted vasa vasorum precede the apparent pathological features of disease [5, 17, 25–28].

4.3 Vasa Vasorum Dysfunction During Disease Initiation

First hypothesized by Karl Köster (1876) [13], Emanuel Aufrecht (1908) [29], and Hippolyte Martin (1881) [30], the idea that vasa vasorum disruption can lead to atherosclerosis development has been around a long time. Obstruction, hypoperfusion, or endothelial barrier leakiness can disrupt the function of vasa vasorum. Because they are **functional end arteries, each vasa vasorum supplies nutrients and oxygen to a confined subintimal area.** This makes the vasa vasorum of the arterial wall especially susceptible to hypoxia as no collateral flow from neighboring vasa vasorum can be expected in case of ischemia or occlusion.

There is abundant evidence that obstruction of vasa vasorum can initiate disease in the parent vessel. Karl Köster (1876) was the first to observe that obstruction of vasa vasorum leads to necrosis of the tunica media and suggested this as an important mechanism in the initiation of atherosclerosis [13]. It was later shown, through microembolism experiments that the obstruction of vasa vasorum did indeed result in vascular lesion development (Fig. 4.3a) [31]. In the case of syphilitic aortitis, spirochaetes have been repeatedly found inside the aortic wall resulting

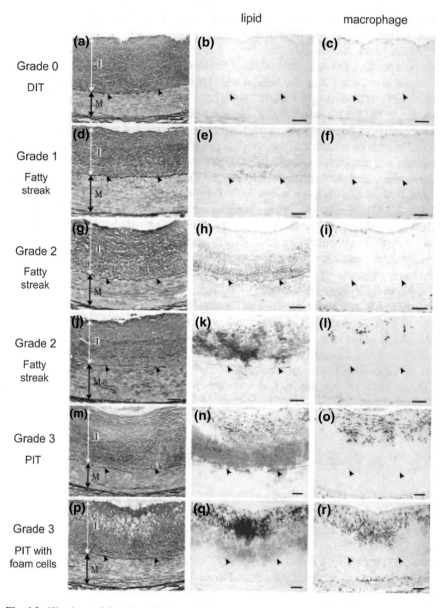

Fig. 4.2 Histology of deposited lipids and infiltrating macrophages into the arterial wall during early atherosclerosis development in humans. Note that lipids are first deposited deep in the intimal layer away from the endothelial layer. Arrowheads indicate internal elastic lamina separating the intima (I) from the media (M). Scale bars represent 100 μm. Reproduced from [24]

in inflammatory obstruction of vasa vasorum [32–34]. In this case, local vessel wall ischemia results in necrosis, focal calcification, and aneurysm formation.

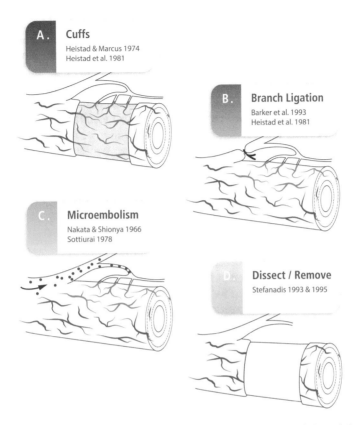

Fig. 4.3 Experimental methods that obstruct or disrupt vasa vasorum perfusion of the arterial wall lead to atherosclerosis in the parent vessel. Exemplary papers demonstrating, **a** obstruction of vasa vasorum by microembolism, **b** constriction of vasa vasorum using arterial cuffs, **c** prevention of vasa vasorum perfusion by ligation of their source branch, and **d** removal of adventitial vasa vasorum

Further experiments that used constriction of vasa vasorum with perivascular cuffs (Fig. 4.3b) or ligation of the arterial branches that supply them (Fig. 4.3c) uniformly produced atherosclerotic lesions in the descending aorta of dogs [35, 36], the femoral artery of pigs [37], and in the carotid artery of rabbits [38]. **These pathological findings were reversible upon removal of the cuff, suggesting structural reversibility of the early manifestations of atherosclerosis.**

In a surgical setting, there is also evidence that vasa vasorum disruption leads to an accelerated atherosclerotic process. Shortly after the first successful human coronary bypass procedure using an autologous saphenous vein as conduit, Brody and colleagues published a detailed histological description of the pathological changes that occur in canine grafts over time [39]. Endothelial damage and thrombosis were primarily restricted to the first postoperative week, during which time the muscular media uniformly displayed extensive necrosis and inflammatory cell infiltration. Brody concluded that these medial changes were initiated by vascular wall ischemia due to interruption of vasa vasorum during transplantation, and only afterward did intimal thickening by myointimal cells and collagen deposition reduce the graft lumen. Margaret Billingham did some of the first and best human pathologic studies of heart transplant patients who died of chronic rejection and transplant coronary artery sclerosis [40–42]. Aortic anastomosis between the organ donor and recipient often revealed normal aortic wall architecture in the recipient segment and severe atherosclerosis in the donor portion of the aorta, implicating damaged and occluded vasa vasorum in graft failure. With the introduction of the "no touch" technique, vein grafts can be harvested with minimal handling of the vessel which is excised with its pedicle of surrounding tissue, including an intact adventitial layer [43]. This technique improves patency compared to conventional harvesting techniques primarily due to the fact that adventitial integrity, and hence vasa vasorum, is preserved.

In a fetus, the ductus arteriosus is a blood vessel connecting the main pulmonary artery to the proximal descending aorta, thereby diverting a major proportion of the right ventricular output away from the pulmonary vascular bed to the umbilical–placental circulation [44]. The ductus arteriosus normally closes in the first few days of life after constriction and, in an accelerated atherosclerosis-like process, anatomic occlusion of the lumen. In premature babies, the ductus arteriosus consists of a thin-layered arterial wall that can be surgically easily clipped. If not, it is occluded in older babies, its wall is severely thickened by "atherosclerotic" debris and, if still open in adults, it is usually calcified. The normal process of occlusion has been closely observed in sheep whereby vasa vasorum hypoperfusion after constriction is responsible for medial hypoxia and subsequent vessel remodeling [45].

In dogs, the functional effects of surgically removing vasa vasorum from the ascending aorta were investigated (Fig. 4.3d) [46, 47]. Compared to the control group, aortic distensibility acutely decreased indicating hypoxia of the wall, and medial necrosis and alterations of the elastin fibers were observed. Thus, both anatomic and functional parameters of blood vessel wall ischemia, as initiated by vasa vasorum dysfunction, could be proven. An increase in vasa vasorum tone, leading to a decrease in microvessel diameter, would result in impaired perfusion and subsequent local hypoxia. There is evidence that plaque-associated vasa vasorum are often poorly perfused [48].

Another significant way vasa vasorum function can be compromised is through leakiness. Angiogenesis is the process of blood vessel sprouting from preexisting vessels. Neovessel formation is triggered primarily in response to hypoxia and/or inflammatory signals. Neovessels, in general, are inherently immature, fragile, and leaky. Arterial vasa vasorum neovascularization is highly correlated with plaque progression and vasa vasorum neovessels show evidence of immaturity and incomplete cellular junctions, with poor mural pericyte coverage [48–51]. As an atherosclerotic plaque progresses, neoangiogenesis continues in an (often futile) effort to maintain sufficient oxygenation of the increasingly hypoxic plaque.

A number of other findings suggest that vasa vasorum neovessels are leaky and serve as conduits for the deposition of atherogenic substances and delivery of inflammatory cells into the parental blood vessel wall. Zhang and colleagues showed that plaque vasa vasorum density and the leakage of plasma components into the arterial wall are connected [52]. Red blood cell (RBC) membranes are rich in cholesterol and the extent of RBC leakage through the vasa vasorum endothelium is hypothesized to significantly contribute to early lipid deposition and later expansion of the necrotic plaque core. In the context of Nakashima's previously mentioned study, permeable vasa vasorum may significantly contribute to the delivery of lipoproteins into the inner layers of the vessel wall. We also have recent evidence that plaque vasa vasorum are leaky. Using old ApoE$^{-/-}$ mice with significant plaque burden, we performed corrosion casting of the arterial system. Electron microscopy of the vasa vasorum within a plaque showed significant leakiness and signs of damage compared to the vasa vasorum adjacent to the plaque (Fig. 4.4).

Vasa vasorum neovascularization is highly correlated with the severity of inflammation within the plaque [23, 49, 53]. Intravital imaging of atherosclerotic mice revealed that vasa vasorum are the main sites where leukocytes enter the plaques [48, 54]. By inhibiting plaque neovascularization, macrophage accumulation in plaques is reduced and plaque progression is slowed down [55]. Critical work in the mid-1990s demonstrated that neovessels express a significantly higher amount of cell adhesion molecules (CAMs), e.g., vascular cell adhesion molecule-1, intercellular adhesion molecule 1, and E-selectin, compared to the luminal endothelium [56–58]. Thus, these studies significantly contributed to our understanding of the mechanism through which vasa vasorum are the primary conduits responsible for leukocyte infiltration into the plaque.

The formation of microvessels in atherosclerotic plaques causes lesions to progress, which increases the risk of rupture [51]. It was shown in ApoE-deficient mice that plaque-associated vasa vasorum are actively angiogenic and perfused [48]. In addition, they are hyperpermeable, have reduced blood flow and blood flow velocity, and demonstrate increased leukocyte adhesion and transmigration. These features promote lesion progression as well as instability, and there is a link to vasa vasorum density. Using human autopsy specimens, Moreno and colleagues compared fibrocalcific and lipid-rich lesions to ruptured plaques [53]. They found increased microvessel density in ruptured plaques. The fibrous caps also demonstrated enhanced vasa vasorum. At the same time, they saw an increase in severity of inflammation. The microvessel density was twice as high in plaques considered vulnerable than in stable ones and four times as high in those that had ruptured [59]. In advanced lesions, the vasa vasorum density is similar in the adventitia and the plaques [60]. Vulnerable plaques display intraplaque hemorrhage, which also promotes instability and complications [61]. A study in ApoE-deficient mice showed that elastin fragmentation in combination with an extremely high-fat diet was associated with plaque instability and rupture [62].

Altogether, we propose that if vasa vasorum become occluded either through mechanical forces or by microthrombi, local microinfarctions of the vessel wall

Fig. 4.4 Electron microscopy of an arterial corrosion cast performed on an 11-month-old ApoE$^{-/-}$ mouse showing the vasa vasorum of the ascending aorta adjacent to (**a**) and within (**b, c**) an atherosclerotic plaque. Interplaque vasa vasorum show significant leakiness. Images courtesy of Nodir Madrahimov (Hannover Medical School)

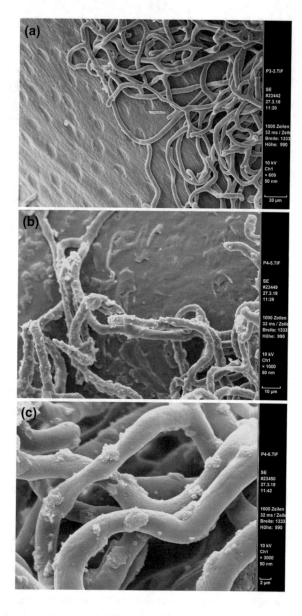

will initiate inflammation, cell necrosis, compensatory hypertrophy, and subsequent "fatty degeneration" [63] of cells leading to plaque formation. Furthermore, systemic or local inflammation in the artery wall as well as hypoxia (e.g., due to occluded vasa vasorum) could lead to leakiness of existing vasa vasorum or the generation of leaky neovessels. Leakiness would contribute to the accumulation of atherogenic factors into the vessel wall, thereby exacerbating site-specific inflammation and plaque formation (Fig. 4.5).

Fig. 4.5 Vasa vasorum
obstruction or malperfusion
leads to localized hypoxia
and necrosis within the
artery wall. Hypoxia or
inflammation induces
angiogenesis and subsequent
leakiness of vasa vasorum.
Leaky vasa vasorum can lead
to deposition of atherogenic
substances in the vessel
wall, contributing to plaque
formation

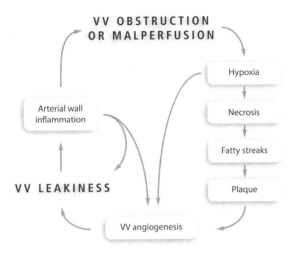

4.4   The Involvement of Vasa Vasorum in Aortic Aneurysms and Dissections

Like atherosclerosis, the pathogenesis of arterial aneurysms remains poorly under-stood. One common theory is that atherosclerosis precipitates arterial aneurysms where it is thought that the atherosclerotic inflammatory processes result in degen-eration of the arterial vessel wall, resulting in aneurysm formation. On the other hand, there are a number of studies providing evidence that the diseases are sep-arate entities which often simply develop in parallel [64]. Supporting this idea is the fact that the presence of atherosclerosis is neither necessary nor sufficient for arterial aneurysm formation [65]. The two diseases also show different predilec-tion sites with arterial aneurysms being most common in the abdominal and tho-racic aorta while being extremely rare in the atherosclerosis-prone sites such as the coronary arteries, the carotid arteries, the superficial femoral arteries, and the aortic arch.

There is sufficient evidence to postulate a similar pathomechanism in arte-rial aneurysm and plaque development. First, arterial aneurysms and athero-sclerosis share many common risk factors and often occur as comorbid conditions. Old age, the male gender, smoking, hypertension, and a familial disposition are all risk factors for the development of arterial aneurysms [66]. In the special case of mycotic aneurysms, which also affect younger patients, infection is also a risk factor for disease development. Similar to acute cardiovascular and cerebrovascu-lar events, aneurysm rupture also shows seasonal variation [67, 68]. A large study with 19,599 patients found there was seasonal variation with a highly significant correlation between cold winter weather and the incidence of aneurysm rupture [67]. The authors speculated that this could be due to the increase in blood pres-sure observed in the winter [69–72] and/or the increased exposure to indoor air pollution, especially tobacco smoke. Supporting the effect of air pollution on arterial aneurysm are experiments on ApoE[-/-] mice where exposure to small particle air pollution significantly increases abdominal aortic aneurysm formation [73]. We would also propose seasonal infections (e.g., influenza, pneumococcal infection) could also play a role in the seasonal variation of arterial aneurysm complications, but this has not been proven to date.

When considering aneurysms, we first need to separate those with a clear hereditary component from sporadic cases. Familial thoracic aortic aneurysm and dissection occur in younger patients with connective tissue disorders, where typical risk factors for "atherosclerotic aneurysms" are not present. In those cases, non-inflammatory media degeneration due to loss of smooth muscle cells and elastic fiber fragmentation results in cystic medial necrosis. In addition, patients with bicuspid aortic valves and/or aortic ischemic sclerosis can also develop non-inflammatory aneurysm in the thoracic aorta. Here as well, however, the function of the aortic wall is genetically diminished regarding its elasticity.

In sporadic (non-hereditary) aneurysm formation, similar to atherosclerosis, increased inflammatory burden on the vessel wall is emerging as a key mechanism in the pathophysiology of disease [74]. In our own experience (unpublished data), screening pathology specimens of subjects following elective ascending thoracic aortic replacement for chronic aneurysms, we were able to detect inflammatory infiltrates in the medial layer of the excised aortic wall in 46 of 72 specimens. Where atherosclerosis and aneurysm formation differ, however, is in the differential expression of cytokines in the affected arterial segments. While immune cells in atherosclerotic plaques primarily express Th1 cytokines, aneurysmal tissue is predominated by a Th2 immune response [75]. From immunohistological studies on elective aneurysm surgery specimens, **aneurysmatic aortae have significantly more activated T-cells and macrophages in the media compared to non-diseased controls** [76–78]. These inflammatory cells are postulated to contribute to the elimination of smooth muscle cells and degeneration of the matrix associated with aneurysm and dissection. Interestingly, infiltration of inflammatory cells is especially seen surrounding the adventitial vasa vasorum, whose endothelial cells also showed increased expression of leukocyte adhesion molecules [76, 77]. This suggests the vasa vasorum at sites of aneurysm formation have an inflamed phenotype and are a conduit for inflammatory cell migration into the media.

There is increasing evidence that vasa vasorum dysfunction is the common link between atherosclerosis and aneurysm formation. Both in animal experiments and human specimens, vasa vasorum occlusion appears to precipitate aneurysm formation. In human abdominal and thoracic aortic aneurysms, stenosis of vasa vasorum in the dilated aortic segments has been observed [79, 80] Accordingly, ischemia or malnutrition of the aortic media due to dysfunctional vasa vasorum can precipitate medial inflammation, degeneration of the aortic wall, and consequently aneurysm formation. This pathomechanism is supported by animal experiments whereby vasa vasorum hypoperfusion in rats leads to aneurysm formation with strikingly similar histopathology to human disease [81]. In addition to vasa vasorum obstruction, there is also evidence of vasa vasorum angiogenesis, remodeling, and leakage in human aneurysms [78, 82]. Thus, there is sufficient evidence to postulate a similar pathomechanism between arterial plaque development and arterial aneurysm.

We will now turn our focus to the similarities between the pathogenesis of atherosclerosis and arterial dissection, which was also historically considered to be initiated in the intima. In 1931, Tyson, a pathologist from Yale, published a series of case reports on aortic dissection, where a number did not show evidence of an intimal tear [83]. In 1953, Hirst and colleagues reviewed the autopsy findings in 505 cases of aortic dissection and found that 4% had no identifiable intimal tear [84]. Based on these and a growing number of similar pathological findings by others, a new hypothesis began to gain favor: that the initiating event in aortic dissection was primary hemorrhage in the media from leakage or rupture of vasa vasorum [85, 86]. Extensive histopathological analyses have demonstrated that most (95%) aortic tears originate in the outer third of the media, alongside the vasa vasorum [85]. In most cases, but not all, this would lead to the subsequent development of a secondary tear of the intima overlying the hemorrhage (Fig. 4.6).

Similar to the inside-out and outside-in theories of atherosclerosis, there are two primary theories on the pathogenesis of aortic and peripheral artery dissection. Both theories were laid out in the 2018 position papers on spontaneous coronary artery dissection from the American Heart Association and the European Cardiology Association [87, 88]. It is still hotly debated whether the causal event is the development of an intimal tear allowing blood to accumulate in the media (inside-out) or whether the causal event is the primary disruption of vasa vasorum leading to hemorrhage directly into the tunica media (outside-in). We would argue

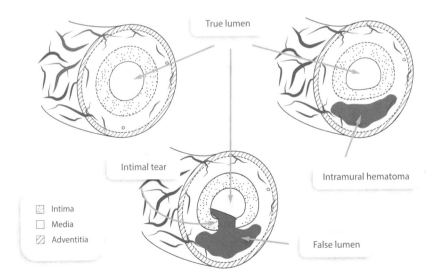

Fig. 4.6 Cross-sectional view of the development of a spontaneous coronary artery dissection. **a** Normal artery, **b** intramural hemorrhage due to disruption of vasa vasorum, **c** dissection with or without an intimal tear

that the observation of intramural hematomas without intimal tears clearly points toward an outside-in mechanism of disease in arterial dissections.

While atherosclerosis and sporadic (non-hereditary) aneurysms occur most often in older individuals, younger and more often female patients are affected by arterial dissection. Similar to the acute events of atherosclerosis (stroke, myocardial infarction), there is significant seasonal variation in aortic and cervical artery dissections [89–92]. Stress and systemic inflammatory disease are also shared risk factors for both atherosclerosis and dissections.

Pathophysiologically, atherosclerosis, aneurysm, and dissections only affect large- and medium-sized arteries where vasa vasorum are prevalent. We strongly believe the unifying observation of malfunctioning vasa vasorum in all three disease entities cannot be overlooked. The inflammatory nature of atherosclerosis may also be operative in both aneurysm formation and aortic/peripheral artery dissection. Older histologic studies as well as recent investigations suggest the medial layer of the artery represents the *locus minoris resistentiae* in all three disease entities with vasa vasorum dysfunction playing a major role. This would clearly support an outside-in concept for the most common phenotypes of arterial disease in surgical practice. Thus, the adventitial layer—that is, the outside of the arterial wall—appears to be the origin of these pathologies with the microcirculation-dependent nutrition and drainage of the arterial wall common denominators of disease initiation and progression. In turn, this notion would imply the tunica intima of the parent vessel to represent the most innocent layer in the arterial wall in these disease processes. If this concept can be supported by further clinical and animal model studies, diagnostic, preventive, and therapeutic measures could focus on the testing, prevention, and restoration of microvascular function in future medicine practice.

4.5   Lymphatic Dysfunction During Atherosclerosis Development

The presence and function of blood vessel wall lymphatics is an understudied and often overlooked aspect of the pathophysiology of atherosclerosis development. Drozdz and colleagues characterized the presence of an extensive lymphatic capillary network in the adventitia of large arteries in humans [93, 94]. The distribution of vessel wall lymphatics follows a similar pattern to vasa vasorum. While primarily in the adventitia, some groups have observed lymphatic vessels in the media and intima of atherosclerotic plaques in both humans and in mouse models of atherosclerosis [95, 96]. In ApoE$^{-/-}$ mice, Taher and colleagues observed that intimal lymphatics in atherosclerotic lesions demonstrate an atypical phenotype [96]. In contrast to adventitial lymphatic vessels, intimal lymphatic vessels did not express lymphatic vessel endothelial hyaluronan receptor 1 (LYVE1) or prospero homeobox protein 1 (PROX1). This unique expression pattern of intimal lymphatic vessels may explain why other groups did not observe lymphatic vessels in the media or intimal before [97, 98]. Similar to vasa vasorum, lymphatic vessels are not uniformly distributed throughout the vascular tree and they increase in density along with atherosclerosis progression [93]. Perhaps it is not surprising that vasa vasorum and lymphatics capillary expansion go hand in hand since angiogenic and lymphangiogenic stimuli overlap. For example, pro-angiogenic growth factors such as vascular endothelial growth factor (VEGF)-A and leukocyte adhesion molecules such as ICAM-1 are involved in the angiogenesis of both vascular systems [99–101]. It has also been suggested that arteries covered by a dense network of lymphatic vessels appear to be protected against atherosclerosis when compared with those that lack such a network [102]. For example, intramural coronary arteries demonstrate a dense plexus of myocardial lymphatic vessels [103]. Therefore, this area is well drained, which may be one reason it is rarely affected by atherosclerosis. In contrast, the absence of lymphatic drainage of the epicardial coronary arteries could predispose them to vessel inflammation [98]. So there seems to be an inverse relationship between the presence of sufficient lymphatic drainage of the arterial wall and the development of atherosclerosis [102].

Local disturbances to lymphatic function also correlate with atherosclerosis development. **Interestingly, if the lymphatic network is damaged as in heart transplantation, smaller coronary arteries and veins that are normally spared become susceptible to atherosclerosis** [103]. In addition, lymphatic blockade results in an increase in intimal thickness in dogs [104] and humans [105]. There is also evidence that, similar to vasa vasorum, the function of lymphatic vessels present in atherosclerosis plaques is compromised [102]. While lymphatic vessels are crucial in clearance of inflammatory mediators, inflammation itself can negatively affect lymphatic function [106, 107]. Arterial wall lymphatic dysfunction would hinder the drainage of lipids, growth factors, inflammatory cytokines, and immune cells. This in turn would affect lymph composition, thereby influencing lymphatic function, homeostasis, tissue pressure, and macrophage retention [108]. Indeed, studies in mice have shown reduced monocyte-derived cell emigration in progressive atherosclerotic lesions [109]. Consequently, insufficient lymphatic drainage of the arterial wall is gaining recognition for its contribution to atherosclerosis development. Importantly, lymphatics are involved in reverse cholesterol transport (RCT) and therefore clearance of cholesterol from the arterial wall [110]. In experiments in mice, Martel and colleagues demonstrated that surgical as well as genetic disruption of lymphatic drainage led to impaired macrophage RCT [110]. In addition, they showed that lymphatic vessels of the aortic wall mediate RCT. Aortae of donor atherosclerotic ApoE-deficient mice with labeled cholesterol were transplanted into recipient ApoE-deficient mice pretreated with anti-VEGFR-3, which blocks lymphatic regrowth. The disrupted RCT led to retention of the labeled cholesterol from the donor proving the role of the lymphatic vasculature. Therefore, impaired lymphatic vessel function leads to increased levels of retained cholesterol within the arterial wall and consequently contributes to atherosclerosis. This was further demonstrated in a study using two transgenic mouse strains with lymphatic insufficiency that were crossed with atherosclerotic mice [111]. These mice showed impaired lipoprotein transport and accumulation of cholesterol in their arteries. In addition, lesions progressed faster in young and intermediate age mice compared to controls. Emigration of monocyte-derived cells from atherosclerotic lesions was impaired leading to retention and reduced clearance of monocytes [109]. Correspondingly, regressing lesions demonstrated migration of these cells from atherosclerotic plaques.

Given their importance in fluid balance, RCT, and the immune system, the underappreciated role of lymphatics is gaining recognition. New preventative and therapeutic approaches to improve lymphatic function, and hence optimize drainage of the arterial wall, are of increasing interest.

References

1. Delewi R, Yang H, Kastelein J. Atherosclerosis. 2013. www.textbookofcardiology.org/wiki/Atherosclerosis. Accessed 4 Jan 2018.
2. Taggart DP. Current status of arterial grafts for coronary artery bypass grafting. Ann Cardiothorac Surg. 2013;2:427–30. https://doi.org/10.3978/j.issn.2225-319X.2013.07.21.
3. Otsuka F, Yahagi K, Sakakura K, Virmani R. Why is the mammary artery so special and what protects it from atherosclerosis? Ann Cardiothorac Surg. 2013;2:519–26. https://doi.org/10.3978/2416.
4. Hildebrandt HA, Gossl M, Mannheim D, et al. Differential distribution of vasa vasorum in different vascular beds in humans. Atherosclerosis. 2008;199:47–54. https://doi.org/10.1016/j.atherosclerosis.2007.09.015.
5. Galili O, Herrmann J, Woodrum J, et al. Adventitial vasa vasorum heterogeneity among different vascular beds. J Vasc Surg. 2004;40:529–35. https://doi.org/10.1016/j.jvs.2004.06.032.
6. Sano M, Unno N, Sasaki T, et al. Topologic distributions of vasa vasorum and lymphatic vasa vasorum in the aortic adventitia-Implications for the prevalence of aortic diseases. Atherosclerosis. 2016;247:127–34. https://doi.org/10.1016/j.atherosclerosis.2016.02.007.
7. Gössl M, Versari D, Mannheim D, et al. Increased spatial vasa vasorum density in the proximal LAD in hypercholesterolemia-Implications for vulnerable plaque-development. Atherosclerosis. 2007;192:246–52. https://doi.org/10.1016/j.atherosclerosis.2006.07.004.
8. Mulligan-Kehoe MJ. The vasa vasorum in diseased and nondiseased arteries. AJP Hear Circ Physiol. 2010;298:H295–305. https://doi.org/10.1152/ajpheart.00884.2009.
9. Kampschulte M, Brinkmann A, Stieger P, et al. Quantitative CT imaging of the spatio-temporal distribution patterns of vasa vasorum in aortas of ApoE$^{-/-}$/LDL$^{-/-}$ double knockout mice. Atherosclerosis. 2010;212:444–50. https://doi.org/10.1016/j.atherosclerosis.2010.07.010.
10. Nishimiya K, Matsumoto Y, Wang H, et al. Absence of adventitial vasa vasorum formation at the coronary segment with myocardial bridge-An optical coherence tomography study. Int J Cardiol. 2018;250:275–7. https://doi.org/10.1016/j.ijcard.2017.09.211.
11. Langheinrich AC, Michniewicz A, Bohle RM, Ritman EL. Vasa vasorum neovascularization and lesion distribution among different vascular beds in ApoE$^{-/-}$/LDL$^{-/-}$ double knockout mice. Atherosclerosis. 2007;191:73–81. https://doi.org/10.1016/j.atherosclerosis.2006.05.021.
12. Langheinrich AC, Michniewicz A, Sedding DG, et al. Correlation of vasa vasorum neovascularization and plaque progression in aortas of apolipoprotein E$^{-/-}$/low-density lipoprotein$^{-/-}$ double knockout mice. Arterioscler Thromb Vasc Biol. 2006;26:347–52. https://doi.org/10.1161/01.ATV.0000196565.38679.6d.

13. Köster K. Endarteritis and Arteritis. Berl Klin Wochenschrift. 1876;13:454–5.
14. Robertson HP. Vascularization of the thoracic aorta. Arch Path. 1929;8:881.
15. Galili O, Sattler KJ, Herrmann J, et al. Experimental hypercholesterolemia differentially affects adventitial vasa vasorum and vessel structure of the left internal thoracic and coronary arteries. J Thorac Cardiovasc Surg. 2005;129:767–72. https://doi.org/10.1016/j.jtcvs.2004.08.014.
16. Clarke JA. An x-ray microscopic study of the blood-supply to the aortic bifurcation and common iliac arteries. Br J Surg. 1966;53:354–8.
17. Geiringer E. Intimal vascularisation and artherosclerosis. J Pathol Bacteriol. 1951;63:201–11. https://doi.org/10.1002/path.1700630204.
18. Kumamoto M, Nakashima Y, Sueishi K. Intimal neovascularization in human coronary atherosclerosis: its origin and pathophysiological significance. Hum Pathol. 1995;26:450–6.
19. van Dijk RA, Virmani R, von der Thüsen JH, et al. The natural history of aortic atherosclerosis: a systematic histopathological evaluation of the peri-renal region. Atherosclerosis. 2010;210:100–6. https://doi.org/10.1016/j.atherosclerosis.2009.11.016.
20. Uchida Y. Recent advances in fluorescent angioscopy for molecular imaging of human atherosclerotic coronary plaque. J Atheroscler Thromb. 2017. https://doi.org/10.5551/jat.40352.
21. Nakashima Y, Wight TN, Sueishi K. Early atherosclerosis in humans: role of diffuse intimal thickening and extracellular matrix proteoglycans. Cardiovasc Res. 2008;79:14–23. https://doi.org/10.1093/cvr/cvn099.
22. Maiellaro K, Taylor W. The role of the adventitia in vascular inflammation. Cardiovasc Res. 2007;75:640–8. https://doi.org/10.1016/j.cardiores.2007.06.023.
23. Boyle EC, Sedding DG, Haverich A. Targeting vasa vasorum dysfunction to prevent atherosclerosis. Vascul Pharmacol. 2017;96–98:5–10. https://doi.org/10.1016/j.vph.2017.08.003.
24. Nakashima Y, Fujii H, Sumiyoshi S, et al. Early human atherosclerosis: accumulation of lipid and proteoglycans in intimal thickenings followed by macrophage infiltration. Arterioscler Thromb Vasc Biol. 2007;27:1159–65. https://doi.org/10.1161/ATVBAHA.106.134080.
25. Herrmann J, Lerman LO, Rodriguez-Porcel M, et al. Coronary vasa vasorum neovascularization precedes epicardial endothelial dysfunction in experimental hypercholesterolemia. Cardiovasc Res. 2001;51:762–6.
26. Häkkinen T, Karkola K, Ylä-Herttuala S. Macrophages, smooth muscle cells, endothelial cells, and T-cells express CD40 and CD40L in fatty streaks and more advanced human atherosclerotic lesions. Colocalization with epitopes of oxidized low-density lipoprotein, scavenger receptor, and CD16 (Fc gammaRIII). Virchows Arch. 2000;437:396–405.
27. Ylä-Herttuala S, Bentzon JF, Daemen M, et al. Stabilisation of atherosclerotic plaques. Position paper of the European Society of Cardiology (ESC) Working Group on atherosclerosis and vascular biology. Thromb Haemost. 2011;106:1–19. https://doi.org/10.1160/TH10-12-0784.
28. Zhu X-Y. Antioxidant intervention attenuates myocardial neovascularization in hypercholesterolemia. Circulation. 2004;109:2109–15. https://doi.org/10.1161/01.CIR.0000125742.65841.8B.
29. Aufrecht E. Die Genese der Arteriosklerose (Arteriitis). Deu Arch f klin Med. 1908;93:1–14.
30. Martin H. Recherches sur la nature et la pathogénie des lésions viscérales consécutives à l'endartérite oblitérante et progressive. Scléroses dystrophiques. Rev méd. 1881;1:369.
31. Nakata Y, Shionoya S. Vascular lesions due to obstruction of the vasa vasorum. Nature. 1966;212:1258–9.
32. Reuter K. Neue befunde von Spirochaeta Pallida in menschlichen Körper und ihre Bedeutung für die Aetiologie der Syphilis. Zeitschrift für Hyg und Infekt. 1906;54:49–60.

33. O'Regan AW, Castro C, Lukehart SA, et al. Barking up the wrong tree? Use of polymerase chain reaction to diagnose syphilitic aortitis. Thorax. 2002;57:917–8.
34. Stone JR, Bruneval P, Angelini A, et al. Consensus statement on surgical pathology of the aorta from the Society for Cardiovascular Pathology and the Association for European Cardiovascular Pathology: I. Inflammatory diseases. Cardiovasc Pathol. 2015;24:267–78. https://doi.org/10.1016/j.carpath.2015.05.001.
35. Heistad DD, Marcus ML. Role of vasa vasorum in nourishment of the aorta. Blood Vessel. 1979;16:225–38.
36. Heistad DD, Marcus ML, Larsen GE, Armstrong ML. Role of vasa vasorum in nourishment of the aortic wall. Am J Physiol. 1981;240:H781–7.
37. Barker SG, Talbert A, Cottam S, et al. Arterial intimal hyperplasia after occlusion of the adventitial vasa vasorum in the pig. Arterioscler Thromb Vasc Biol. 1993;13:70–7. https://doi.org/10.1161/01.ATV.13.1.70.
38. Booth RFG, Martin JF, Honey AC, et al. Rapid development of atherosclerotic lesions in the rabbit carotid artery induced by perivascular manipulation. Atherosclerosis. 1989;76:257–68. https://doi.org/10.1016/0021-9150(89)90109-3.
39. Brody WR, Angeli WW, Kosek JC. Histologic fate of the venous coronary artery bypass in dogs. Am J Pathol. 1972;66:111–30.
40. Billingham ME. Endomyocardial biopsy diagnosis of acute rejection in cardiac allografts. Prog Cardiovasc Dis. 1990;33:11–8.
41. Fujita M, Russell ME, Masek MA, et al. Graft vascular disease in the great vessels and vasa vasorum. Hum Pathol. 1993;24:1067–72.
42. Caves PK, Stinson EB, Billingham ME, et al. Diagnosis of human cardiac allograft rejection by serial cardiac biopsy. J Thorac Cardiovasc Surg. 1973;66:461–6.
43. Barner HB, Farkas EA. Conduits for coronary bypass: vein grafts. Korean J Thorac Cardiovasc Surg. 2012;45:275–86. https://doi.org/10.5090/kjtcs.2012.45.5.275.
44. Gournay V. The ductus arteriosus: physiology, regulation, and functional and congenital anomalies. Arch Cardiovasc Dis. 2011;104:578–85. https://doi.org/10.1016/j.acvd.2010.06.006.
45. Kajino H, Goldbarg S, Roman C, et al. Vasa vasorum hypoperfusion is responsible for medial hypoxia and anatomic remodeling in the newborn lamb ductus arteriosus. Pediatr Res. 2002;51:228–35. https://doi.org/10.1203/00006450-200202000-00017.
46. Stefanadis CI, Karayannacos PE, Boudoulas HK, et al. Medial necrosis and acute alterations in aortic distensibility following removal of the vasa vasorum of canine ascending aorta. Cardiovasc Res. 1993;27:951–6.
47. Stefanadis C, Vlachopoulos C, Karayannacos P, et al. Effect of vasa vasorum flow on structure and function of the aorta in experimental animals. Circulation. 1995;91:2669–78.
48. Rademakers T, Douma K, Hackeng TM, et al. Plaque-associated vasa vasorum in aged apolipoprotein E-deficient mice exhibit proatherogenic functional features in vivo. Arterioscler Thromb Vasc Biol. 2013;33:249–56. https://doi.org/10.1161/ATVBAHA.112.300087.
49. Jeziorska M, Woolley DE. Neovascularization in early atherosclerotic lesions of human carotid arteries: its potential contribution to plaque development. Hum Pathol. 1999;30:919–25.
50. Dunmore BJ, McCarthy MJ, Naylor AR, Brindle NPJ. Carotid plaque instability and ischemic symptoms are linked to immaturity of microvessels within plaques. J Vasc Surg. 2007;45:155–9. https://doi.org/10.1016/j.jvs.2006.08.072.
51. Sluimer JC, Daemen MJ. Novel concepts in atherogenesis: angiogenesis and hypoxia in atherosclerosis. J Pathol. 2009;218:7–29. https://doi.org/10.1002/path.2518.
52. Zhang Y, Cliff WJ, Schoefl GI, Higgins G. Immunohistochemical study of intimal microvessels in coronary atherosclerosis. Am J Pathol. 1993;143:164–72.

53. Moreno PR, Purushothaman KR, Fuster V, et al. Plaque neovascularization is increased in ruptured atherosclerotic lesions of human aorta: implications for plaque vulnerability. Circulation. 2004;110:2032–8. https://doi.org/10.1161/01.CIR.0000143233.87854.23.

54. Eriksson EE. Intravital microscopy on atherosclerosis in apolipoprotein e-deficient mice establishes microvessels as major entry pathways for leukocytes to advanced lesions. Circulation. 2011;124:2129–38. https://doi.org/10.1161/CIRCULATIONAHA.111.030627.

55. Moulton KS, Vakili K, Zurakowski D, et al. Inhibition of plaque neovascularization reduces macrophage accumulation and progression of advanced atherosclerosis. Proc Natl Acad Sci. 2003;100:4736–41. https://doi.org/10.1073/pnas.0730843100.

56. Nakashima Y, Raines EW, Plump AS, et al. Upregulation of VCAM-1 and ICAM-1 at atherosclerosis-prone sites on the endothelium in the ApoE-deficient mouse. Arterioscler Thromb Vasc Biol. 1998;18:842–51.

57. Skinner SA, O'Brien PE. The microvascular structure of the normal colon in rats and humans. J Surg Res. 1996;61:482–90. https://doi.org/10.1006/jsre.1996.0151.

58. O'Brien KD, Allen MD, McDonald TO, et al. Vascular cell adhesion molecule-1 is expressed in human coronary atherosclerotic plaques. Implications for the mode of progression of advanced coronary atherosclerosis. J Clin Invest. 1993;92:945–51. https://doi.org/10.1172/JCI116670.

59. Virmani R, Kolodgie FD, Burke AP, et al. Atherosclerotic plaque progression and vulnerability to rupture: angiogenesis as a source of intraplaque hemorrhage. Arterioscler Thromb Vasc Biol. 2005;25:2054–61. https://doi.org/10.1161/01.ATV.0000178991.71605.18.

60. Sluimer JC, Kolodgie FD, Bijnens APJJ, et al. Thin-walled microvessels in human coronary atherosclerotic plaques show incomplete endothelial junctions. J Am Coll Cardiol. 2009;53:1517–27. https://doi.org/10.1016/j.jacc.2008.12.056.

61. Michel J-B, Virmani R, Arbustini E, Pasterkamp G. Intraplaque haemorrhages as the trigger of plaque vulnerability. Eur Heart J. 2011;32:1977–85. https://doi.org/10.1093/eurheartj/ehr054.

62. Van der Donckt C, Van Herck JL, Schrijvers DM, et al. Elastin fragmentation in atherosclerotic mice leads to intraplaque neovascularization, plaque rupture, myocardial infarction, stroke, and sudden death. Eur Heart J. 2015;36:1049–58. https://doi.org/10.1093/eurheartj/ehu041.

63. Virchow R. Die Cellularpathologie in ihrer Begründung auf physiologische und pathologische Gewebelehre. Berlin: Hirschwald; 1858.

64. Johnsen SH, Forsdahl SH, Singh K, Jacobsen BK. Atherosclerosis in abdominal aortic aneurysms: a causal event or a process running in parallel? The Tromsø study. Arterioscler Thromb Vasc Biol. 2010;30:1263–8. https://doi.org/10.1161/ATVBAHA.110.203588.

65. Sterpetti AV, Feldhaus RJ, Schultz RD, Blair EA. Identification of abdominal aortic aneurysm patients with different clinical features and clinical outcomes. Am J Surg. 1988;156:466–9.

66. Peshkova IO, Schaefer G, Koltsova EK. Atherosclerosis and aortic aneurysm-is inflammation a common denominator? FEBS J. 2016;283:1636–52. https://doi.org/10.1111/febs.13634.

67. Ballaro A, Cortina-Borja M, Collin J. A seasonal variation in the incidence of ruptured abdominal aortic aneurysms. Eur J Vasc Endovasc Surg. 1998;15:429–31.

68. Xie N, Zou L, Ye L. The effect of meteorological conditions and air pollution on the occurrence of type A and B acute aortic dissections. Int J Biometeorol. 2018;62:1607–13. https://doi.org/10.1007/s00484-018-1560-0.

69. Brennan PJ, Greenberg G, Miall WE, Thompson SG. Seasonal variation in arterial blood pressure. Br Med J (Clin Res Ed). 1982;285:919–23.

70. Hata T, Ogihara T, Maruyama A, et al. The seasonal variation of blood pressure in patients with essential hypertension. Clin Exp Hypertens A. 1982;4:341–54.

71. Imai Y, Munakata M, Tsuji I, et al. Seasonal variation in blood pressure in normotensive women studied by home measurements. Clin Sci (Lond). 1996;90:55–60.

72. Iwahori T, Miura K, Obayashi K, et al. Seasonal variation in home blood pressure: findings from nationwide web-based monitoring in Japan. BMJ Open. 2018;8:e017351. https://doi.org/10.1136/bmjopen-2017-017351.

73. Jun X, Jin G, Fu C, et al. PM2.5 promotes abdominal aortic aneurysm formation in angiotensin II-infused apoe$^{-/-}$ mice. Biomed Pharmacother. 2018;104:550–7. https://doi.org/10.1016/j.biopha.2018.04.107.

74. Pisano C, Balistreri CR, Ricasoli A, Ruvolo G. Cardiovascular disease in ageing: an overview on thoracic aortic aneurysm as an emerging inflammatory disease. Mediators Inflamm. 2017;2017:1274034. https://doi.org/10.1155/2017/1274034.

75. Schönbeck U, Sukhova GK, Gerdes N, Libby P. T(H)2 predominant immune responses prevail in human abdominal aortic aneurysm. Am J Pathol. 2002;161:499–506. https://doi.org/10.1016/S0002-9440(10)64206-X.

76. He R, Guo D-C, Estrera AL, et al. Characterization of the inflammatory and apoptotic cells in the aortas of patients with ascending thoracic aortic aneurysms and dissections. J Thorac Cardiovasc Surg. 2006;131:671–8. https://doi.org/10.1016/j.jtcvs.2005.09.018.

77. He R, Guo D-C, Sun W, et al. Characterization of the inflammatory cells in ascending thoracic aortic aneurysms in patients with Marfan syndrome, familial thoracic aortic aneurysms, and sporadic aneurysms. J Thorac Cardiovasc Surg. 2008;136(922–9):929.e1. https://doi.org/10.1016/j.jtcvs.2007.12.063.

78. Billaud M, Hill JC, Richards TD, et al. Medial hypoxia and adventitial vasa vasorum remodeling in human ascending aortic aneurysm. Front Cardiovasc Med. 2018;5:124. https://doi.org/10.3389/fcvm.2018.00124.

79. Guo D-C, Pannu H, Tran-Fadulu V, et al. Mutations in smooth muscle alpha-actin (ACTA2) lead to thoracic aortic aneurysms and dissections. Nat Genet. 2007;39:1488–93. https://doi.org/10.1038/ng.2007.6.

80. Tanaka H, Zaima N, Sasaki T, et al. Adventitial vasa vasorum arteriosclerosis in abdominal aortic aneurysm. PLoS One. 2013;8:e57398. https://doi.org/10.1371/journal.pone.0057398.

81. Tanaka H, Zaima N, Sasaki T, et al. Hypoperfusion of the adventitial vasa vasorum develops an abdominal aortic aneurysm. PLoS One. 2015;10:e0134386. https://doi.org/10.1371/journal.pone.0134386.

82. Kessler K, Borges LF, Ho-Tin-Noé B, et al. Angiogenesis and remodelling in human thoracic aortic aneurysms. Cardiovasc Res. 2014;104:147–59. https://doi.org/10.1093/cvr/cvu196.

83. Tyson MD. Dissecting aneurysms. Am J Pathol. 1931;7(581–604):13.

84. Hirst AE, Johns VJ, Kime SW. Dissecting aneurysm of the aorta: a review of 505 cases. Med (Baltimore). 1958;37:217–79.

85. Osada H, Kyogoku M, Ishidou M, et al. Aortic dissection in the outer third of the media: what is the role of the vasa vasorum in the triggering process? Eur J Cardiothorac Surg. 2013;43:e82–8. https://doi.org/10.1093/ejcts/ezs640.

86. Völker W, Dittrich R, Grewe S, et al. The outer arterial wall layers are primarily affected in spontaneous cervical artery dissection. Neurology. 2011;76:1463–71. https://doi.org/10.1212/WNL.0b013e318217e71c.

87. Hayes SN, Kim ESH, Saw J, et al. Spontaneous coronary artery dissection: current state of the science: a scientific statement from the American heart association. Circulation. 2018;137:e523–57. https://doi.org/10.1161/CIR.0000000000000564.

88. Adlam D, Alfonso F, Maas A, et al. European Society of Cardiology, acute cardiovascular care association, SCAD study group: a position paper on spontaneous coronary artery dissection. Eur Heart J. 2018;39:3353–68. https://doi.org/10.1093/eurheartj/ehy080.

89. Thomas LC, Hall LA, Attia JR, et al. Seasonal variation in spontaneous cervical artery dissection: comparing between UK and Australian sites. J Stroke Cerebrovasc Dis. 2017;26:177–85. https://doi.org/10.1016/j.jstrokecerebrovasdis.2016.09.006.

90. Thomas LC, Makaroff AP, Oldmeadow C, et al. Seasonal variation in cervical artery dissection in the Hunter New England region, New South Wales, Australia: a retrospective cohort study. Musculoskelet Sci Pract. 2017;27:106–11. https://doi.org/10.1016/j.math.2016.10.007.

91. Takagi H, Ando T, Umemoto T, (ALICE [All-Literature Investigation of Cardiovascular Evidence] Group). Meta-analysis of seasonal incidence of aortic dissection. Am J Cardiol. 2017;120:700–7. https://doi.org/10.1016/j.amjcard.2017.05.040.

92. Vitale J, Manfredini R, Gallerani M, et al. Chronobiology of acute aortic rupture or dissection: a systematic review and a meta-analysis of the literature. Chronobiol Int. 2015;32:385–94. https://doi.org/10.3109/07420528.2014.983604.

93. Drozdz K, Janczak D, Dziegiel P, et al. Adventitial lymphatics of internal carotid artery in healthy and atherosclerotic vessels. Folia Histochem Cytobiol. 2008;46:433–6. https://doi.org/10.2478/v10042-008-0083-7.

94. Drozdz K, Janczak D, Dziegiel P, et al. Adventitial lymphatics and atherosclerosis. Lymphology. 2012;45:26–33.

95. Kholová I, Dragneva G, Čermáková P, et al. Lymphatic vasculature is increased in heart valves, ischaemic and inflamed hearts and in cholesterol-rich and calcified atherosclerotic lesions. Eur J Clin Invest. 2011;41:487–97. https://doi.org/10.1111/j.1365-2362.2010.02431.x.

96. Taher M, Nakao S, Zandi S, et al. Phenotypic transformation of intimal and adventitial lymphatics in atherosclerosis: a regulatory role for soluble VEGF receptor 2. FASEB J. 2016;30:2490–9. https://doi.org/10.1096/fj.201500112.

97. Nakano T, Nakashima Y, Yonemitsu Y, et al. Angiogenesis and lymphangiogenesis and expression of lymphangiogenic factors in the atherosclerotic intima of human coronary arteries. Hum Pathol. 2005;36:330–40. https://doi.org/10.1016/j.humpath.2005.01.001.

98. Eliska O, Eliskova M, Miller AJ. The absence of lymphatics in normal and atherosclerotic coronary arteries in man: a morphologic study. Lymphology. 2006;39:76–83.

99. Doyle B, Caplice N. Plaque neovascularization and antiangiogenic therapy for atherosclerosis. J Am Coll Cardiol. 2007;49:2073–80. https://doi.org/10.1016/j.jacc.2007.01.089.

100. Cueni LN, Detmar M. The lymphatic system in health and disease. Lymphat Res Biol. 2008;6:109–22. https://doi.org/10.1089/lrb.2008.1008.

101. Lorier G, Touriño C, Kalil RAK. Coronary angiogenesis as an endogenous response to myocardial ischemia in adults. Arq Bras Cardiol. 2011;97:e140–8.

102. Kutkut I, Meens MJ, McKee TA, et al. Lymphatic vessels: an emerging actor in atherosclerotic plaque development. Eur J Clin Invest. 2015;45:100–8. https://doi.org/10.1111/eci.12372.

103. Miller AJ, DeBoer A, Palmer A. The role of the lymphatic system in coronary atherosclerosis. Med Hypotheses. 1992;37:31–6.

104. Nádasy GL, Solti F, Monos E, et al. Effect of two week lymphatic occlusion on the mechanical properties of dog femoral arteries. Atherosclerosis. 1989;78:251–60.

105. Nakata Y, Shionoya S. Structure of lymphatics in the aorta and the periaortic tissues, and vascular lesions caused by disturbance of the lymphatics. Lymphology. 1979;12:18–9.

106. Aldrich MB, Sevick-Muraca EM. Cytokines are systemic effectors of lymphatic function in acute inflammation. Cytokine. 2013;64:362–9. https://doi.org/10.1016/j.cyto.2013.05.015.

107. Zawieja DC, Greiner ST, Davis KL, et al. Reactive oxygen metabolites inhibit spontaneous lymphatic contractions. Am J Physiol. 1991;260:H1935–43. https://doi.org/10.1152/ajpheart.1991.260.6.H1935.

108. Milasan A, Ledoux J, Martel C. Lymphatic network in atherosclerosis: the underestimated path. Futur Sci OA. 2015;1:FSO61. https://doi.org/10.4155/fso.15.61.

109. Llodra J, Angeli V, Liu J, et al. Emigration of monocyte-derived cells from atherosclerotic lesions characterizes regressive, but not progressive, plaques. Proc Natl Acad Sci USA. 2004;101:11779–84. https://doi.org/10.1073/pnas.0403259101.

110. Martel C, Li W, Fulp B, et al. Lymphatic vasculature mediates macrophage reverse choles-
     terol transport in mice. J Clin Invest. 2013;123:1571–9. https://doi.org/10.1172/JCI63685.
111. Vuorio T, Nurmi H, Moulton K, et al. lymphatic vessel insufficiency in hypercholester-
     olemic mice alters lipoprotein levels and promotes atherogenesis. Arterioscler Thromb
     Vasc Biol. 2014;34:1162–70. https://doi.org/10.1161/ATVBAHA.114.302528.

Chapter 5
Risk Factors and Prevention in Light of Atherosclerosis Being a Microvascular Disease

5.1 General

The entire endothelium of an adult human is estimated to cover over $1000 \, m^2$ [1]. The majority of endothelial cells in the body are within the microvasculature while the larger conduit arteries and veins are covered by only a few square meters of endothelial cells. Therefore, it should not come as a surprise that microvessels play a fundamental role in the regulation of the cardiovascular system and to the homeostasis of body organs.

If one considers atherosclerosis a disease initiated in the vessel wall microvasculature, associated risk factors truly start to make sense. Vasa vasorum dysfunction can occur through obstruction or malperfusion, both of which result in vessel wall hypoxia. Hypoxia-driven neoangiogenesis generates leaky microvessels which subsequently allow inflammatory substances into the vessel wall, driving more inflammation-induced endothelial leakiness. We believe that vasa vasorum obstruction and/or leakage contribute to localized inflammation and cell death, precipitating site-specific, vasa vasorum-dependent plaque formation (Fig. 5.1). In this chapter, we will examine how risk factors might contribute to vasa vasorum dysfunction and how the vasa vasorum could be key targets of the beneficial actions of current preventative therapies.

5.2 How Risk Factors Affect the Microcirculation

Obstruction of vasa vasorum may be the result of microthrombosis. Many atherosclerosis risk factors result in a hemostatic balance that leans toward a pro-thrombotic/pro-coagulant state. Let's start with aging—the most dominant risk factor for clinically relevant disease. Aging is strongly associated with a pro-coagulant state

© Springer Nature Switzerland AG 2019
A. Haverich and E. C. Boyle, *Atherosclerosis Pathogenesis and Microvascular Dysfunction*, https://doi.org/10.1007/978-3-030-20245-3_5

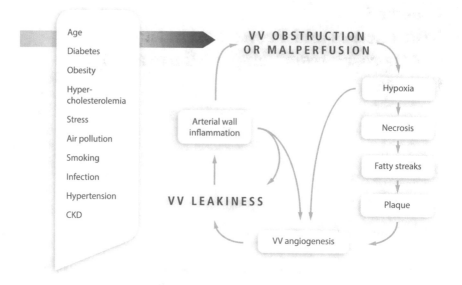

Fig. 5.1 Atherosclerosis risk factors precipitate vasa vasorum dysfunction. Vasa vasorum obstruction or malperfusion leads to localized hypoxia and necrosis within the artery wall. Hypoxia or inflammation induces angiogenesis and subsequent leakiness of vasa vasorum. Leaky vasa vasorum can lead to deposition of atherogenic substances in the vessel wall, contributing to plaque formation

and predisposition to thrombosis [2, 3]. While platelet counts decrease slightly with age, functionally they show signs of abnormal activation [4–7]. von Willebrand factor (vWF) is a large multimeric glycoprotein that mediates the adhesion and aggregation of platelets to sites of vascular injury. vWF levels in the plasma increase with age and are associated with pathological thrombosis [8–10]. Elevated vWF levels are also associated with hypertension [11, 12], hypercholesterolemia [13, 14], diabetes [15–17], obesity [11, 18, 19], and chronic kidney disease [20]—all important risk factors for atherosclerosis and conditions which exhibit a hypercoagulable state. Hypercoagulation associated with polycythemia vera results in coronary microvascular dysfunction, thereby contributing to the higher risk of cardiovascular disease in individuals with this disease [21].

Emotional stress is a well known yet relatively underappreciated risk factor for cardiovascular events [22]. In humans, an intriguing study here in Germany found an association between watching a major sporting event (World Cup soccer) and a higher risk of myocardial infarction [23]. **We propose the mechanistic link between stress and atherosclerosis lies in the effect of stress hormones on the vasa vasorum.** Epinephrine (adrenaline) is known to induce thrombus formation [24] and could therefore result in obstruction of vasa vasorum. Mental stress is also known to cause vasoconstriction of the microvasculature [25–27] and in this way could lead to mechanical constriction of vasa vasorum. And lastly, uptake of LDL into arterial walls has been observed in response to noradrenaline and adrenaline in both rabbits and rats [28–30]. Therefore, through obstruction, malperfusion, and/or leakiness, stress may cause vasa vasorum dysfunction which likely contributes to atherosclerosis development and acute cardiovascular events.

In addition, microthrombosis can arise from neutrophil extracellular traps (NETs)—highly condensed DNA structures released from neutrophils which are covered in antimicrobial peptides. While the release of NETs (NETosis) is an important innate immune defense that can trap and kill pathogens [31], they also can have pro-thrombotic consequences. NETs are released by activated neutrophils during infection, hypoxia, or inflammation, and cause platelet adhesion, aggregation, and activation [32, 33]. In turn, activated platelets further trigger NETosis [34]. NETs have been detected in atherosclerotic lesions and in arterial thrombi in both humans and mice and have been suggested to play a causative role in triggering plaque formation [35–39]. Interestingly, many atherosclerosis risk factors are associated with an increase in NETosis. With age, neutrophil numbers increase [40], NETosis increases [41], and platelets are abnormally activated. Therefore, with age, the stage is set for NET-induced thrombosis and the potential obstruction of vasa vasorum. Oxidized LDL [42], cholesterol crystals [35], cigarette smoking [43], and obesity [44] all trigger NETosis. Patients with end-stage renal disease and on dialysis also demonstrate increased levels of NETosis [45]. Moreover, increasing evidence shows a strong link between NETosis and both type 1 and 2 diabetes [46–48]. Elevated glucose, homocysteine, and hyperglycemia in type 2 diabetes are associated with the release of NETs and the anti-diabetic drug metformin reduces NETosis [49]. Therefore, we hypothesize that age—together with any additional insults like infection or other risk factors that cause systemic inflammation—amplifies NETosis thereby potentiating vasa vasorum obstruction and contributing to the initiation of atherosclerosis.

Increasingly, exposure to particulate matter (PM) air pollution is considered a significant risk factor for atherosclerosis as well as other diseases associated with microcirculatory disturbances such as diabetes [50–54] and dementia [55–57]. Data from animal models and controlled exposure studies in man support the fact that PM exposure results in a pro-thrombotic state [58]. Mechanistically, the majority of evidence suggest that this occurs through activation of platelets, while inflammatory and oxidative stress also seem to contribute to the PM-induced pro-coagulant/thrombotic state [59–67].

This brings us nicely to the link between ABO blood groups, air pollution, and cardiovascular disease incidence. Several large studies have reported the influence of blood type on plasma concentrations of the blood clotting protein vWF, with group O individuals having lower vWF levels than non-O individuals [68–72]. More recently, several studies correlated the non-O blood group with an increased incidence of cardiovascular disease [73–75]. At the 2017 Heart Failure meeting, a meta-analysis of over 1.3 million individuals was presented, including 11 prospective cohorts in nine peer-reviewed papers [76]. They found that non-O blood groups had a 9% increased risk of coronary or cardiovascular events. Together, these studies suggest that non-O blood increases thrombotic risk. Intriguingly, it was also reported that non-O blood type individuals are at higher risk of PM2.5-induced cardiovascular events [77]. Therefore, the picture becomes clearer—**non-O blood type individuals have higher vWF levels putting them at higher risk** of (PM-, infection-, and age-induced) microthrombi of the vasa vasorum, and hence at higher risk of atherosclerosis and the associated cardiovascular events.

Mechanistically, how the microbiota could affect atherosclerosis development is beginning to be understood (Fig. 5.2). In mice, the intestinal microbiota has been shown to modulate synthesis of serotonin which in turn has a pro-thrombotic effect on platelets [78]. The intestinal microbiota was also discovered to be a potential environmental determinant of plasma vWF levels [79]. Germ-free mice were shown to have much lower levels of vWF than conventionally raised mice. Furthermore, enhanced vWF expression, which occurred specifically in liver endothelial cells, required microbiota-triggered toll-like receptor-2 (TLR2) signaling. Importantly, the effect of the intestinal microbiota on plasma vWF levels translated to significant differences in arterial thrombus formation. Whether these findings will translate to humans is currently not known but raises the exciting possibility that an individual's serotonin and vWF levels can be modulated by external, possibly modifiable factors.

The diet- and microbiota-dependent metabolite TMAO is an emerging risk factor in the development of cardiovascular disease and there is increasing mechanistic evidence that the association might be causal. TMAO has been shown to increase thrombosis formation by directly altering calcium signaling in platelets, leading to platelet aggregation [80, 81]. TMAO also promotes vascular inflammation through activation of NF-kB signaling in endothelial and smooth muscle cells [82]. Therefore, elevated systemic TMAO could affect the vasa vasorum microvasculature through both microthrombosis- and inflammation-induced dysfunction. Interestingly, elevated TMAO is not only associated with atherosclerosis but also other diseases (and comorbidities) such as chronic kidney disease, type 2 diabetes, and nonalcoholic fatty liver disease (reviewed by [83]). We hypothesize that the underlying pathomechanism linking elevated TMAO to these diseases involves its effect on the microvasculature.

While coagulant/thrombotic obstruction of vasa vasorum clearly leads to localized hypoxia, constriction or compression leading to vasa vasorum malperfusion can also cause hypoxia of the surrounding vessel wall. How might atherosclerosis risk factors like aging, obesity, smoking, air pollution, and diabetes contribute to constriction or compression of vasa vasorum? Systemic oxidative stress and inflammation that occurs as a result of exposure to many risk factors causes an imbalance in vascular homeostasis that favors vasoconstriction. In controlled exposure experiments in humans, nicotine and particulate air pollution cause vasoconstriction of peripheral small vessels [84, 85]. Aging and obesity share numerous pathophysiologies with each being associated with elevated plasma concentrations of the hormone endothelin-1 (ET-1), a potent vasoconstrictor [86–88]. Elevated ET-1 is associated with age- and obesity-related diminished endothelial vasodilator capacity and enhanced vasoconstrictor tone [87, 89–91]. Accordingly, increasing ET-1 levels which correlate with increasing age and adiposity likely

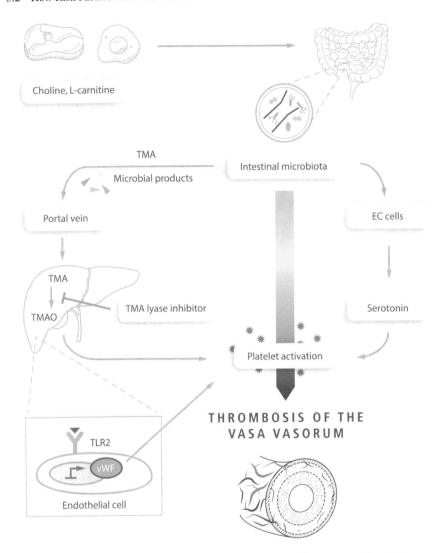

Fig. 5.2 Multiple ways in which the intestinal microbiota can affect the arterial wall microvasculature. Intestinal microbiota influences the number and function of enterochromaffin (EC) cells thereby promoting the release of serotonin. Serotonin, in turn, increases platelet activation. Choline and L-carnitine from the diet get converted to trimethylamine (TMA) by the gut microbiota. In the liver, TMA is metabolized to trimethylamine-N-oxide (TMAO) which directly activates platelets and stimulates inflammatory signaling in the endothelium. Gut microbial products also regulate hepatic von Willebrand factor (vWF) synthesis and arterial thrombus formation via toll-like receptor-2 (TLR2)

lead to constriction of vasa vasorum. Other studies have shown that risk factors contribute to increased vascular ET-1 activity. In controlled exposure experiments in humans, diesel PM did not increase the plasma levels of ET-1 but increased vascular sensitivity to vasoconstrictive effects of ET-1 [92]. An increase in ET-1-dependent vasoconstrictor tone has also been reported for hypertension [93], hypercholesterolemia [94], and type 2 diabetes mellitus [95]. Because vasa vasorum are end arteries and because the effects of vasoconstriction are highest in small vessels, vasa vasorum would be especially susceptible to risk-factor-induced vasoconstriction. Importantly, almost all of the major atherosclerosis risk factors raise blood pressure. With increasing blood pressure, blood flow through vasa vasorum can be compromised due to the compressive forces on the arterial wall (according to Lame's law). **Therefore, hypertension would cause malperfusion of vasa vasorum and hypoxia in especially the microvessels away from the adventitia.** Altogether, we have made a strong case for impaired microcirculation being a unifying factor underlying many atherosclerosis risk factors.

5.3   How Risk Factors Affect Endothelial Repair and Regeneration

Both circulating and vascular resident stem/progenitor cells play a critical role in maintaining the structural and functional integrity of the endothelium in the face of injury as well as provide the building blocks for angiogenesis [96, 97]. The level of bone-marrow-derived circulating endothelial progenitor cells (EPCs) correlates with and is an independent predictor of cardiovascular disease [98–100]. Many atherosclerosis risk factors have detrimental effects on the number and/or function of EPCs, including exposure to PM air pollution [101–103], obesity [104], diabetes [105, 106], smoking, hypertension, age, and LDL cholesterol [107]. In fact, the number and migratory activity of circulating EPCs is inversely correlated with the total number of risk factors an individual possesses [98, 107]. This is thought to occur through increased levels of reactive oxygen species (ROS) and inflammation [108, 109]. The generation of ROS in particular has especially potent effects on stem/progenitor cell migration, proliferation, and differentiation (reviewed by [110]). Because of their potential role in regeneration, repair, and angiogenesis, EPCs could play an important role in preventing risk-factor-induced vasa vasorum dysfunction [111].

The blood vessel wall itself is also a reservoir of resident EPCs and it is becoming increasingly clear that these resident cells have the ability to respond to injury and contribute to endothelial repair (reviewed by [112]). For example, prompted by certain growth factors or inflammatory cytokines in the microenvironment, Sca-1+ resident vascular progenitor cells can differentiate into endothelial cells, participate in regeneration of the vascular endothelium, and promote atherosclerosis plaque stabilization [113, 114]. The effect of risk factors (hypertension, hyperlipidemia, smoking, obesity) on resident EPCs is just beginning to be investigated but it seems likely that excess risk-factor-induced reactive oxygen species production also leads to defects in resident EPC proliferation and differentiation [96, 112, 115].

5.4 Common Preventative Measures and Therapies Affecting the Microvasculature

Lifestyle modifications are a major way to prevent atherosclerosis. Diabetics are recommended to closely manage their blood glucose levels, smokers are counseled to quit, and overweight/inactive individuals are given dietary recommendations and are encouraged to begin an exercise regime. As part of primary or secondary prevention, patients are given anti-hypertensive (e.g., ACE inhibitors, beta-blockers, ET-1 receptor antagonists), anti-thrombotic (e.g., low-dose aspirin, thrombin receptor agonists), and lipid-lowering drugs (e.g., statins) (Table 5.1). And due to the results of the CANTOS trial, anti-inflammatory drugs will likely soon be adopted into the standard of care. Anti-oxidant vitamins (e.g., C, D, E) have beneficial effects on endothelial function and can lower inflammatory cytokines circulating the blood [116–118]. Therefore, at risk, patients are often encouraged to ingest more anti-oxidants. We would argue that much of what cardiologists recommend today for prevention and treatment of atherosclerosis (i.e., drugs and lifestyle modifications) may relate to previously unrecognized benefits to the vasa vasorum microvasculature.

Statins are potent inhibitors of cholesterol biosynthesis and are the most widely prescribed drugs in the world. Let's consider how statins might affect the vasa vasorum. First, lowering serum cholesterol levels would reduce the amount of cholesterol available to be deposited in the vessel wall via leaky vasa vasorum. In addition, as cholesterol crystals are triggers of NETosis, statins would also prevent NET-induced microthrombi from forming in the vasa vasorum. Independent of their lipid-lowering ability, statins also have numerous pleiotropic effects, most prominently anti-inflammatory properties. Many large studies have looked at how statins reduce serum levels of CRP [135–139]—a systemic marker of inflammation and independent predictor of atherosclerosis risk. Patients with low CRP levels after statin therapy have better clinical outcomes than those with higher CRP levels, regardless of LDL cholesterol levels in the blood [140]. This strongly suggests that the ability of statins to reduce inflammation is central to their ability to prevent atherosclerosis. Ultimately, less systemic inflammation would mean less maladaptive vasa vasorum angiogenesis and less NET-based vasa vasorum microthrombi.

The microcirculation is now considered an important target for statins' anti-oxidative, anti-inflammatory, and anti-thrombogenic effects [141, 142]. NO regulates vessel tone [143], maintains a non-thrombotic endothelial surface [144], and reduces leukocyte–endothelium interactions [145]. Statins increase the production of endothelial NO [146, 147], reduce the production of reactive oxygen species that would quench NO [148], and reduce ET-1 levels [149]. Statins would thereby increase blood flow by dilating vasa vasorum. Statins also inhibit leukocyte–endothelium interactions primarily through downregulation of cell adhesion molecular expression [150–152] or blocking CAMs themselves [153]. And through their effects on post-translation modification of small GTPases,

Table 5.1 Cardiovascular disease drug therapies (adapted from [119])

Class	Drug	Examples	Mechanism of action	Reference
Anti-thrombotic	Thromboxane inhibitors	Aspirin, triflusal	Platelet COX-1 inhibitors	[120, 121]
		Terutroban	Thromboxane receptor antagonist	
	ADP P2Y receptor antagonists	Thienopyridines (e.g., clopidogrel, prasugrel)	Bind irreversibly to ADP $P2Y_{12}$ ADP receptors	[122–124]
		Non-thienopyridines (e.g., ticagrelor, cangrelor)	Bind reversibly to $P2Y_{12}$ ADP receptors; active drug	
	GPIIb/IIIa inhibitors	Abciximab	Monoclonal antibody that irreversibly blocks GPIIb/IIIa receptors	[125]
		Eptifibatide, tirofiban	Synthetic molecules that reversibly bind GPIIa/IIIb receptors	
	Thrombin receptor antagonists	Varopaxar, atopaxar	Platelet thrombin receptor antagonist	[126]
	vWF-GPIb inhibitors*	AJW200, 82D6A3	Prevent vWF-GPIb interaction by inhibiting platelet adhesion	[127]
	Nitric oxide-donating aspirin derivative*	NCX-4016	NO donor+platelet COX-1 inhibition	[128]
	Soluble CD39*	solCD39	ATP and ADP metabolization	[129]
Anti-hypertensive	Beta-blocker	Propranolol, Bisoprolol	Block action of catecholamines on beta-adrenergic receptors	[130]
	Endothelin receptor antagonist	Darusentan	Block action of endothelin	[131]
	ACE inhibitors	Ramipril, lisinopril	Activation of RAS system	[132]
Anti-inflammatory	Statins	Atorvastatin	Upregulates eNOS	[133]
	Monoclonal antibodies	Canakinumab	Antibody against IL-1β	[134]

*Under investigation or development

statins result in cytoskeletal stability of the endothelial junctions, thereby reducing inflammation-induced leakiness [154]. Therefore, through inhibition of cell adhesion molecules and maintenance of microvascular tone and endothelial barrier integrity, statins have important beneficial effects on vasa vasorum structure and function. Statins also influence platelet function, altering their activation, and ultimately reducing platelet thrombus formation [133, 155–157]. As a consequence, we hypothesize that less vasa vasorum obstruction would occur when on statins and therefore atherosclerosis development would be hampered.

Statin therapy can also affect endothelial progenitor cells and their ability to regenerate the vasculature [158]. Short-term statin use increases the number of circulating EPCs [107, 159, 160]. However, one study found that long-term statin use is associated with reduced numbers of circulating EPCs [161]. For that reason, it seems statins would have a more or less transient effect on EPC-mediated endothelial repair and angiogenesis and would not resolve prolonged vasa vasorum dysfunction. In the future, it would also be of interest to determine whether statin use affects resident EPC numbers or function.

There is a large body of evidence showing that moderate intensity exercise training is highly effective in improving cardiovascular health in both healthy individuals and ones with preexisting disease [162–165]. Aerobic exercise has favorable effects on several of the traditional risk factors of cardiovascular disease in that it lowers blood pressure [166], reduces adiposity [167–169], and improves serum lipid profiles [170]. However, **much of the benefit of aerobic exercise relates to its positive effects on both macro- and microvascular endothelial function** [171, 172]. Moderate aerobic exercise also results in a significant release of bone-marrow-derived EPCs which home to sites of injury and repair damaged endothelium and provide the building blocks for neoangiogenesis [173–175]. Exercise-induced EPC mobilization would support vasa vasorum regeneration in the face of ischemic or inflammatory damage. The mechanisms underlying the benefits of exercise on the endothelium include suppression of pro-inflammatory cytokine expression [176–178], enhancement of anti-inflammatory mediators and anti-oxidants [179, 180], and promotion of fibrinolytic and DNAse 1 activity [178, 181–183]. Therefore, the effects of exercise protect against microvascular dysfunction induced by risk-factor-induced stressors. And as previously discussed, because the vasa vasorum microvasculature is particularly susceptible to microthrombosis, vasoconstriction, and leakiness due to inflammation, exercise would benefit these small vessels the most. And lastly, exercise increases lymphatic flow [184] and consequently likely supports clearance of atherogenic substances from the arterial wall.

Interestingly, both statin therapy and exercise training have been shown to have positive therapeutic effects in many other disease entities involving the microvasculature including diabetes [185, 186], Alzheimer's/dementia [187–193], cancer [194–197], periodontal disease [198, 199], and nonalcoholic fatty liver disease [200–202]. Many risk factors, including exposure to air pollution, are shared between atherosclerosis and the aforementioned disease entities (Fig. 5.3). The common risk factors and therapies shared between these diseases suggest they

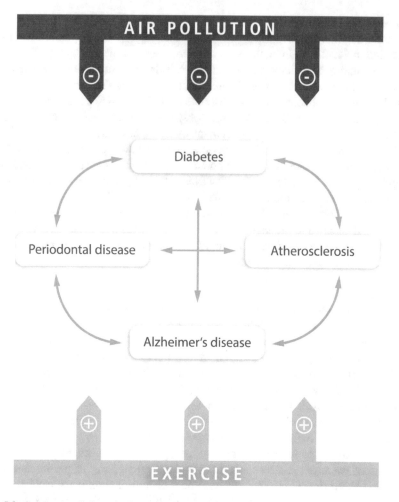

Fig. 5.3 Substantive links exist between different disease entities and they share the common risk factor of air pollution and the common benefit of exercise

may share similar underlying pathomechanisms and support the idea that atherosclerosis is a member of this family of microcirculatory diseases.

References

1. Wolinsky H. A proposal linking clearance of circulating lipoproteins to tissue metabolic activity as a basis for understanding atherogenesis. Circ Res. 1980;47:301–11. https://doi.org/10.1161/01.RES.47.3.301.
2. Sepúlveda C, Palomo I, Fuentes E. Primary and secondary haemostasis changes related to aging. Mech Ageing Dev. 2015;150:46–54. https://doi.org/10.1016/j.mad.2015.08.006.

3. Sepúlveda C, Palomo I, Fuentes E. Mechanisms of endothelial dysfunction during aging: predisposition to thrombosis. Mech Ageing Dev. 2017;164:91–9. https://doi.org/10.1016/j.mad.2017.04.011.

4. Segal JB, Moliterno AR. Platelet counts differ by sex, ethnicity, and age in the United States. Ann Epidemiol. 2006;16:123–30. https://doi.org/10.1016/j.annepidem.2005.06.052.

5. Reilly IAG, FitzGerald GA. Eicosenoid biosynthesis and platelet function with advancing age. Thromb Res. 1986;41:545–54. https://doi.org/10.1016/0049-3848(86)91700-7.

6. Kasjanovová D, Baláz V. Age-related changes in human platelet function in vitro. Mech Ageing Dev. 1986;37:175–82.

7. Zahavi J, Jones NA, Leyton J, et al. Enhanced in vivo platelet "release reaction" in old healthy individuals. Thromb Res. 1980;17:329–36.

8. Conlan MG, Folsom AR, Finch A, et al. Associations of factor VIII and von Willebrand factor with age, race, sex, and risk factors for atherosclerosis. The Atherosclerosis Risk in Communities (ARIC) Study. Thromb Haemost. 1993;70:380–5.

9. Favaloro EJ, Soltani S, McDonald J, et al. Reassessment of ABO blood group, sex, and age on laboratory parameters used to diagnose von Willebrand disorder: potential influence on the diagnosis vs the potential association with risk of thrombosis. Am J Clin Pathol. 2005;124:910–7.

10. Shahidi M. Thrombosis and von Willebrand factor. Adv Exp Med Biol. 2017;906:285–306. https://doi.org/10.1007/5584_2016_122.

11. Blann AD, Bushell D, Davies A, et al. von Willebrand factor, the endothelium and obesity. Int J Obes Relat Metab Disord. 1993;17:723–5.

12. Ma W-H, Sheng L, Gong H-P, et al. The application of vWF/ADAMTS13 in essential hypertension. Int J Clin Exp Med. 2014;7:5636–42.

13. Blann AD, Dobrotova M, Kubisz P, McCollum CN. von Willebrand factor, soluble P-selectin, tissue plasminogen activator and plasminogen activator inhibitor in atherosclerosis. Thromb Haemost. 1995;74:626–30.

14. Blann AD. Assessment of endothelial dysfunction: focus on atherothrombotic disease. Pathophysiol Haemost Thromb. 2003;33:256–61. https://doi.org/10.1159/000083811.

15. Lufkin EG, Fass DN, O'Fallon WM, Bowie EJ. Increased von Willebrand factor in diabetes mellitus. Metabolism. 1979;28:63–6.

16. Kessler L, Wiesel ML, Attali P, et al. Von Willebrand factor in diabetic angiopathy. Diabetes Metab. 1998;24:327–36.

17. Seligman BG, Biolo A, Polanczyk CA, et al. Increased plasma levels of endothelin 1 and von Willebrand factor in patients with type 2 diabetes and dyslipidemia. Diabetes Care. 2000;23:1395–400.

18. Mousa SA. Elevation of plasma von Willebrand factor and tumor necrosis factor-a in obese subjects and their reduction by the low molecular weight heparin tinzaparin. Int Angiol. 2005;24:278–81.

19. Patel SR, Bellary S, Karimzad S, Gherghel D. Overweight status is associated with extensive signs of microvascular dysfunction and cardiovascular risk. Sci Rep. 2016;6:32282. https://doi.org/10.1038/srep32282.

20. Holvoet P, Donck J, Landeloos M, et al. Correlation between oxidized low density lipoproteins and von Willebrand factor in chronic renal failure. Thromb Haemost. 1996;76:663–9.

21. Vianello F, Cella G, Osto E, et al. Coronary microvascular dysfunction due to essential thrombocythemia and policythemia vera: the missing piece in the puzzle of their increased cardiovascular risk? Am J Hematol. 2015;90:109–13. https://doi.org/10.1002/ajh.23881.

22. Chida Y, Steptoe A. Greater cardiovascular responses to laboratory mental stress are associated with poor subsequent cardiovascular risk status: a meta-analysis of prospective evidence. Hypertension. 2010;55:1026–32. https://doi.org/10.1161/HYPERTENSIONAHA.109.146621. (Dallas, Tex 1979).

23. Wilbert-Lampen U, Leistner D, Greven S, et al. Cardiovascular events during World Cup soccer. N Engl J Med. 2008;358:475–83. https://doi.org/10.1056/NEJMoa0707427.

24. Lin H, Young DB. Opposing effects of plasma epinephrine and norepinephrine on coronary thrombosis in vivo. Circulation. 1995;91:1135–42.
25. Ramadan R, Sheps D, Esteves F, et al. Myocardial ischemia during mental stress: role of coronary artery disease burden and vasomotion. J Am Heart Assoc. 2013;2:e000321. https://doi.org/10.1161/JAHA.113.000321.
26. Dakak N, Quyyumi AA, Eisenhofer G, et al. Sympathetically mediated effects of mental stress on the cardiac microcirculation of patients with coronary artery disease. Am J Cardiol. 1995;76:125–30.
27. Arrighi JA, Burg M, Cohen IS, et al. Myocardial blood-flow response during mental stress in patients with coronary artery disease. Lancet (London, England). 2000;356:310–1. https://doi.org/10.1016/S0140-6736(00)02510-1.
28. Born GV, Shafi S, Cusack NJ. Evidence for the acceleration of atherogenesis by circulating norepinephrine. Transplant Proc. 1989;21:3660–1.
29. Shafi S, Cusack NJ, Born GV. Increased uptake of methylated low-density lipoprotein induced by noradrenaline in carotid arteries of anaesthetized rabbits. Proc R Soc Lond Ser B Biol Sci. 1989;235:289–98. https://doi.org/10.1098/rspb.1989.0001.
30. Cardona-Sanclemente LE, Born GV. Adrenaline increases the uptake of low-density lipoproteins in carotid arteries of rabbits. Atherosclerosis. 1992;96:215–8.
31. Brinkmann V, Reichard U, Goosmann C, et al. Neutrophil extracellular traps kill bacteria. Science. 2004;303:1532–5. https://doi.org/10.1126/science.1092385.
32. Demers M, Krause DS, Schatzberg D, et al. Cancers predispose neutrophils to release extracellular DNA traps that contribute to cancer-associated thrombosis. Proc Natl Acad Sci. 2012;109:13076–81. https://doi.org/10.1073/pnas.1200419109.
33. Fuchs TA, Brill A, Duerschmied D, et al. Extracellular DNA traps promote thrombosis. Proc Natl Acad Sci USA. 2010;107:15880–5. https://doi.org/10.1073/pnas.1005743107.
34. Etulain J, Martinod K, Wong SL, et al. P-selectin promotes neutrophil extracellular trap formation in mice. Blood. 2015;126:242–6. https://doi.org/10.1182/blood-2015-01-624023.
35. Warnatsch A, Ioannou M, Wang Q, Papayannopoulos V. Neutrophil extracellular traps license macrophages for cytokine production in atherosclerosis. Science. 2015;349:316–20. https://doi.org/10.1126/science.aaa8064.
36. Megens RTA, Vijayan S, Lievens D, et al. Presence of luminal neutrophil extracellular traps in atherosclerosis. Thromb Haemost. 2012;107:597–8. https://doi.org/10.1160/TH11-09-0650.
37. Riegger J, Byrne RA, Joner M, et al. Histopathological evaluation of thrombus in patients presenting with stent thrombosis. A multicenter European study: a report of the prevention of late stent thrombosis by an interdisciplinary global European effort consortium. Eur Heart J. 2016;37:1538–49. https://doi.org/10.1093/eurheartj/ehv419.
38. de Boer O, Li X, Teeling P, et al. Neutrophils, neutrophil extracellular traps and interleukin-17 associate with the organisation of thrombi in acute myocardial infarction. Thromb Haemost. 2013;109:290–7. https://doi.org/10.1160/TH12-06-0425.
39. Döring Y, Soehnlein O, Weber C. Neutrophil extracellular traps in atherosclerosis and atherothrombosis. Circ Res. 2017;120:736–43. https://doi.org/10.1161/CIRCRESAHA.116.309692.
40. Schröder AK, Rink L. Neutrophil immunity of the elderly. Mech Ageing Dev. 2003;124:419–25.
41. Martinod K, Witsch T, Erpenbeck L, et al. Peptidylarginine deiminase 4 promotes age-related organ fibrosis. J Exp Med. 2017;214:439–58. https://doi.org/10.1084/jem.20160530.
42. Awasthi D, Nagarkoti S, Kumar A, et al. Oxidized LDL induced extracellular trap formation in human neutrophils via TLR-PKC-IRAK-MAPK and NADPH-oxidase activation. Free Radic Biol Med. 2016;93:190–203. https://doi.org/10.1016/j.freeradbiomed.2016.01.004.
43. Qiu S-L, Zhang H, Tang Q-Y, et al. Neutrophil extracellular traps induced by cigarette smoke activate plasmacytoid dendritic cells. Thorax. 2017;72:1084–93. https://doi.org/10.1136/thoraxjnl-2016-209887.

44. Wang H, Wang Q, Venugopal J, et al. Obesity-induced endothelial dysfunction is prevented by neutrophil extracellular trap inhibition. Sci Rep. 2018;8:4881. https://doi.org/10.1038/s41598-018-23256-y.

45. Kim J-K, Hong C-W, Park MJ, et al. Increased neutrophil extracellular trap formation in uremia is associated with chronic inflammation and prevalent coronary artery disease. J Immunol Res. 2017;2017:8415179. https://doi.org/10.1155/2017/8415179.

46. Wang Y, Xiao Y, Zhong L, et al. Increased neutrophil elastase and proteinase 3 and augmented NETosis are closely associated with -cell autoimmunity in patients with type 1 diabetes. Diabetes. 2014;63:4239–48. https://doi.org/10.2337/db14-0480.

47. Menegazzo L, Ciciliot S, Poncina N, et al. NETosis is induced by high glucose and associated with type 2 diabetes. Acta Diabetol. 2015;52:497–503. https://doi.org/10.1007/s00592-014-0676-x.

48. Fadini GP, Menegazzo L, Rigato M, et al. NETosis delays diabetic wound healing in mice and humans. Diabetes. 2016;65:1061–71. https://doi.org/10.2337/db15-0863.

49. Menegazzo L, Scattolini V, Cappellari R, et al. The antidiabetic drug metformin blunts NETosis in vitro and reduces circulating NETosis biomarkers in vivo. Acta Diabetol. 2018;55:593–601. https://doi.org/10.1007/s00592-018-1129-8.

50. Park SK, Adar SD, O'Neill MS, et al. Long-term exposure to air pollution and type 2 diabetes mellitus in a multiethnic cohort. Am J Epidemiol. 2015;181:327–36. https://doi.org/10.1093/aje/kwu280.

51. Krämer U, Herder C, Sugiri D, et al. Traffic-related air pollution and incident type 2 diabetes: results from the SALIA cohort study. Environ Health Perspect. 2010;118:1273–9. https://doi.org/10.1289/ehp.0901689.

52. Weinmayr G, Hennig F, Fuks K, et al. Long-term exposure to fine particulate matter and incidence of type 2 diabetes mellitus in a cohort study: effects of total and traffic-specific air pollution. Environ Heal. 2015;14:53. https://doi.org/10.1186/s12940-015-0031-x.

53. Coogan PF, White LF, Jerrett M, et al. Air pollution and incidence of hypertension and diabetes mellitus in black women living in Los Angeles. Circulation. 2012;125:767–72. https://doi.org/10.1161/CIRCULATIONAHA.111.052753.

54. Clark C, Sbihi H, Tamburic L, et al. Association of long-term exposure to transportation noise and traffic-related air pollution with the incidence of diabetes: a prospective cohort study. Environ Health Perspect. 2017;125:087025. https://doi.org/10.1289/EHP1279.

55. Killin LOJ, Starr JM, Shiue IJ, Russ TC. Environmental risk factors for dementia: a systematic review. BMC Geriatr. 2016;16:175. https://doi.org/10.1186/s12877-016-0342-y.

56. Chen H, Kwong JC, Copes R, et al. Exposure to ambient air pollution and the incidence of dementia: a population-based cohort study. Environ Int. 2017;108:271–7. https://doi.org/10.1016/j.envint.2017.08.020.

57. Tzivian L, Dlugaj M, Winkler A, et al. Long-term air pollution and traffic noise exposures and mild cognitive impairment in older adults: a cross-sectional analysis of the Heinz Nixdorf recall study. Environ Health Perspect. 2016;124:1361–8. https://doi.org/10.1289/ehp.1509824.

58. Robertson S, Miller MR. Ambient air pollution and thrombosis. Part Fibre Toxicol. 2018;15:1. https://doi.org/10.1186/s12989-017-0237-x.

59. Hajat A, Allison M, Diez-Roux AV, et al. Long-term exposure to air pollution and markers of inflammation, coagulation, and endothelial activation: a repeat-measures analysis in the Multi-Ethnic Study of Atherosclerosis (MESA). Epidemiology. 2015;26:310–20. https://doi.org/10.1097/EDE.0000000000000267.

60. Jacobs L, Emmerechts J, Mathieu C, et al. Air pollution related prothrombotic changes in persons with diabetes. Environ Health Perspect. 2010;118:191–6. https://doi.org/10.1289/ehp.0900942.

61. Cozzi E, Wingard CJ, Cascio WE, et al. Effect of ambient particulate matter exposure on hemostasis. Transl Res. 2007;149:324–32. https://doi.org/10.1016/j.trsl.2006.12.009.

62. Radomski A, Jurasz P, Alonso-Escolano D, et al. Nanoparticle-induced platelet aggregation and vascular thrombosis. Br J Pharmacol. 2005;146:882–93. https://doi.org/10.1038/sj.bjp.0706386.

63. Ghio AJ, Hall A, Bassett MA, et al. Exposure to concentrated ambient air particles alters hematologic indices in humans. Inhal Toxicol. 2003;15:1465–78. https://doi.org/10.1080/08958370390249111.
64. Lucking AJ, Lundback M, Mills NL, et al. Diesel exhaust inhalation increases thrombus formation in man. Eur Heart J. 2008;29:3043–51. https://doi.org/10.1093/eurheartj/ehn464.
65. Lucking AJ, Lundbäck M, Barath SL, et al. Particle traps prevent adverse vascular and prothrombotic effects of diesel engine exhaust inhalation in men. Circulation. 2011;123:1721–8. https://doi.org/10.1161/CIRCULATIONAHA.110.987263.
66. Nemmar A, Hoylaerts MF, Hoet PHM, Nemery B. Possible mechanisms of the cardiovascular effects of inhaled particles: systemic translocation and prothrombotic effects. Toxicol Lett. 2004;149:243–53. https://doi.org/10.1016/j.toxlet.2003.12.061.
67. Wu S, Deng F, Wei H, et al. Chemical constituents of ambient particulate air pollution and biomarkers of inflammation, coagulation and homocysteine in healthy adults: a prospective panel study. Part Fibre Toxicol. 2012;9:49. https://doi.org/10.1186/1743-8977-9-49.
68. Franchini M, Capra F, Targher G, et al. Relationship between ABO blood group and von Willebrand factor levels: from biology to clinical implications. Thromb J. 2007;5:14. https://doi.org/10.1186/1477-9560-5-14.
69. Smith NL, Chen M-H, Dehghan A, et al. Novel associations of multiple genetic loci with plasma levels of factor VII, factor VIII, and von Willebrand factor: The CHARGE (Cohorts for Heart and Aging Research in Genome Epidemiology) Consortium. Circulation. 2010;121:1382–92. https://doi.org/10.1161/CIRCULATIONAHA.109.869156.
70. Miller CH, Haff E, Platt SJ, et al. Measurement of von Willebrand factor activity: relative effects of ABO blood type and race. J Thromb Haemost. 2003;1:2191–7.
71. Song J, Chen F, Campos M, et al. Quantitative influence of ABO blood groups on factor VIII and its ratio to von Willebrand factor, novel observations from an ARIC study of 11,673 subjects. PLoS ONE. 2015;10:e0132626. https://doi.org/10.1371/journal.pone.0132626.
72. Gill JC, Endres-Brooks J, Bauer PJ, et al. The effect of ABO blood group on the diagnosis of von Willebrand disease. Blood. 1987;69:1691–5.
73. He M, Wolpin B, Rexrode K, et al. ABO blood group and risk of coronary heart disease in two prospective cohort studies. Arterioscler Thromb Vasc Biol. 2012;32:2314–20. https://doi.org/10.1161/ATVBAHA.112.248757.
74. Wu O, Bayoumi N, Vickers MA, Clark P. ABO(H) blood groups and vascular disease: a systematic review and meta-analysis. J Thromb Haemost. 2008;6:62–9. https://doi.org/10.1111/j.1538-7836.2007.02818.x.
75. Tanis B, Algra A, van der Graaf Y, et al. Procoagulant factors and the risk of myocardial infarction in young women. Eur J Haematol. 2006;77:67–73. https://doi.org/10.1111/j.1600-0609.2006.00656.x.
76. Kole TM, Suthahar N, Damman K, De Boer RA. ABO blood group and cardiovascular outcomes in the general population: a meta-analysis. Eur J Hear Fail. 2017;19:175.
77. Horne BD, Muhlestein JB, Carlquist JF, et al. Interaction of genetic variation in the ABO locus and short-term exposure to elevations in fine particulate matter air pollution differentially affects associations with acute coronary events. Am Hear Assoc Sci Sess Meet Anaheim, CA;2017.
78. Yano JM, Yu K, Donaldson GP, et al. Indigenous bacteria from the gut microbiota regulate host serotonin biosynthesis. Cell. 2015;161:264–76. https://doi.org/10.1016/j.cell.2015.02.047.
79. Jäckel S, Kiouptsi K, Lillich M, et al. Gut microbiota regulate hepatic von Willebrand factor synthesis and arterial thrombus formation via Toll-like receptor-2. Blood. 2017;130:542–53. https://doi.org/10.1182/blood-2016-11-754416.
80. Zhu W, Gregory JC, Org E, et al. Gut microbial metabolite TMAO enhances platelet hyperreactivity and thrombosis risk. Cell. 2016;165:111–24. https://doi.org/10.1016/j.cell.2016.02.011.

81. Zhu W, Wang Z, Tang WHW, Hazen SL. Gut microbe-generated trimethylamine n-oxide from dietary choline is prothrombotic in subjects. Circulation. 2017;135:1671–3. https://doi.org/10.1161/CIRCULATIONAHA.116.025338.

82. Seldin MM, Meng Y, Qi H, et al. Trimethylamine N-Oxide promotes vascular inflammation through signaling of mitogen-activated protein kinase and nuclear factor-κB. J Am Heart Assoc. 2016;5. https://doi.org/10.1161/JAHA.115.002767.

83. Brown JM, Hazen SL. Microbial modulation of cardiovascular disease. Nat Rev Microbiol. 2018;16:171–81. https://doi.org/10.1038/nrmicro.2017.149.

84. Klein LW. Cigarette smoking, atherosclerosis and the coronary hemodynamic response: a unifying hypothesis. J Am Coll Cardiol. 1984;4:972–4.

85. Brook RD, Brook JR, Urch B, et al. Inhalation of fine particulate air pollution and ozone causes acute arterial vasoconstriction in healthy adults. Circulation. 2002;105:1534–6.

86. Goel A, Su B, Flavahan S, et al. Increased endothelial exocytosis and generation of endothelin-1 contributes to constriction of aged arteries. Circ Res. 2010;107:242–51. https://doi.org/10.1161/CIRCRESAHA.109.210229.

87. Donato AJ, Gano LB, Eskurza I, et al. Vascular endothelial dysfunction with aging: endothelin-1 and endothelial nitric oxide synthase. Am J Physiol Heart Circ Physiol. 2009;297:H425–32. https://doi.org/10.1152/ajpheart.00689.2008.

88. Weil BR, Westby CM, Van Guilder GP, et al. Enhanced endothelin-1 system activity with overweight and obesity. Am J Physiol Heart Circ Physiol. 2011;301:H689–95. https://doi.org/10.1152/ajpheart.00206.2011.

89. Westby CM, Weil BR, Greiner JJ, et al. Endothelin-1 vasoconstriction and the age-related decline in endothelium-dependent vasodilatation in men. Clin Sci (Lond). 2011;120:485–91. https://doi.org/10.1042/CS20100475.

90. Van Guilder GP, Stauffer BL, Greiner JJ, Desouza CA. Impaired endothelium-dependent vasodilation in overweight and obese adult humans is not limited to muscarinic receptor agonists. Am J Physiol Heart Circ Physiol. 2008;294:H1685–92. https://doi.org/10.1152/ajpheart.01281.2007.

91. Schinzari F, Iantorno M, Campia U, et al. Vasodilator responses and endothelin-dependent vasoconstriction in metabolically healthy obesity and the metabolic syndrome. Am J Physiol Endocrinol Metab. 2015;309:E787–92. https://doi.org/10.1152/ajpendo.00278.2015.

92. Langrish JP, Lundbäck M, Mills NL, et al. Contribution of endothelin 1 to the vascular effects of diesel exhaust inhalation in humans. Hypertens. 2009;54:910–5. https://doi.org/10.1161/HYPERTENSIONAHA.109.135947. (Dallas, Tex 1979).

93. Cardillo C, Nambi SS, Kilcoyne CM, et al. Insulin stimulates both endothelin and nitric oxide activity in the human forearm. Circulation. 1999;100:820–5.

94. Cardillo C, Kilcoyne CM, Cannon RO, Panza JA. Increased activity of endogenous endothelin in patients with hypercholesterolemia. J Am Coll Cardiol. 2000;36:1483–8.

95. Cardillo C, Campia U, Bryant MB, Panza JA. Increased activity of endogenous endothelin in patients with type II diabetes mellitus. Circulation. 2002;106:1783–7.

96. Xie Y, Fan Y, Xu Q. Vascular regeneration by stem/progenitor cells. Arterioscler Thromb Vasc Biol. 2016;36:e33–40. https://doi.org/10.1161/ATVBAHA.116.307303.

97. Lee PSS, Poh KK. Endothelial progenitor cells in cardiovascular diseases. World J Stem Cells. 2014;6:355–66. https://doi.org/10.4252/wjsc.v6.i3.355.

98. Hill JM, Zalos G, Halcox JPJ, et al. Circulating endothelial progenitor cells, vascular function, and cardiovascular risk. N Engl J Med. 2003;348:593–600. https://doi.org/10.1056/NEJMoa022287.

99. Schmidt-Lucke C, Rössig L, Fichtlscherer S, et al. Reduced number of circulating endothelial progenitor cells predicts future cardiovascular events: proof of concept for the clinical importance of endogenous vascular repair. Circulation. 2005;111:2981–7. https://doi.org/10.1161/CIRCULATIONAHA.104.504340.

100. Werner N, Wassmann S, Ahlers P, et al. Endothelial progenitor cells correlate with endothelial function in patients with coronary artery disease. Basic Res Cardiol. 2007;102:565–71. https://doi.org/10.1007/s00395-007-0680-1.

101. O'Toole TE, Hellmann J, Wheat L, et al. Episodic exposure to fine particulate air pollution decreases circulating levels of endothelial progenitor cells. Circ Res. 2010;107:200–3. https://doi.org/10.1161/CIRCRESAHA.110.222679.

102. Niu J, Liberda EN, Qu S, et al. The role of metal components in the cardiovascular effects of PM2.5. PLoS One. 2013;8:e83782. https://doi.org/10.1371/journal.pone.0083782.

103. Cui Y, Sun Q, Liu Z. Ambient particulate matter exposure and cardiovascular diseases: a focus on progenitor and stem cells. J Cell Mol Med. 2016;20:782–93. https://doi.org/10.1111/jcmm.12822.

104. Heida N-M, Müller J-P, Cheng I-F, et al. Effects of obesity and weight loss on the functional properties of early outgrowth endothelial progenitor cells. J Am Coll Cardiol. 2010;55:357–67. https://doi.org/10.1016/j.jacc.2009.09.031.

105. Tepper OM, Galiano RD, Capla JM, et al. Human endothelial progenitor cells from type II diabetics exhibit impaired proliferation, adhesion, and incorporation into vascular structures. Circulation. 2002;106:2781–6.

106. Fadini GP, Miorin M, Facco M, et al. Circulating endothelial progenitor cells are reduced in peripheral vascular complications of type 2 diabetes mellitus. J Am Coll Cardiol. 2005;45:1449–57. https://doi.org/10.1016/j.jacc.2004.11.067.

107. Vasa M, Fichtlscherer S, Aicher A, et al. Number and migratory activity of circulating endothelial progenitor cells inversely correlate with risk factors for coronary artery disease. Circ Res. 2001;89:E1–7.

108. Aicher A, Heeschen C, Mildner-Rihm C, et al. Essential role of endothelial nitric oxide synthase for mobilization of stem and progenitor cells. Nat Med. 2003;9:1370–6. https://doi.org/10.1038/nm948.

109. Lin C-P, Lin F-Y, Huang P-H, et al. Endothelial progenitor cell dysfunction in cardiovascular diseases: role of reactive oxygen species and inflammation. Biomed Res Int. 2013;2013:845037. https://doi.org/10.1155/2013/845037.

110. Bigarella CL, Liang R, Ghaffari S. Stem cells and the impact of ROS signaling. Development. 2014;141:4206–18. https://doi.org/10.1242/dev.107086.

111. Hu Y, Davison F, Zhang Z, Xu Q. Endothelial replacement and angiogenesis in arteriosclerotic lesions of allografts are contributed by circulating progenitor cells. Circulation. 2003;108:3122–7. https://doi.org/10.1161/01.CIR.0000105722.96112.67.

112. Zhang L, Issa Bhaloo S, Chen T, et al. Role of resident stem cells in vessel formation and arteriosclerosis. Circ Res. 2018;122:1608–24. https://doi.org/10.1161/CIRCRESAHA.118.313058.

113. Wong MM, Chen Y, Margariti A, et al. Macrophages Control vascular stem/progenitor cell plasticity through tumor necrosis factor-α-mediated nuclear factor-κB activation. Arterioscler Thromb Vasc Biol. 2014;34:635–43. https://doi.org/10.1161/ATVBAHA.113.302568.

114. Tsai T-N, Kirton JP, Campagnolo P, et al. Contribution of stem cells to neointimal formation of decellularized vessel grafts in a novel mouse model. Am J Pathol. 2012;181:362–73. https://doi.org/10.1016/j.ajpath.2012.03.021.

115. Torsney E, Xu Q. Resident vascular progenitor cells. J Mol Cell Cardiol. 2011;50:304–11. https://doi.org/10.1016/j.yjmcc.2010.09.006.

116. Tousoulis D, Antoniades C, Tentolouris C, et al. Effects of combined administration of vitamins C and E on reactive hyperemia and inflammatory process in chronic smokers. Atherosclerosis. 2003;170:261–7.

117. van Herpen-Broekmans WMR, Klöpping-Ketelaars IAA, Bots ML, et al. Serum carotenoids and vitamins in relation to markers of endothelial function and inflammation. Eur J Epidemiol. 2004;19:915–21.

118. Rashidi B, Hoseini Z, Sahebkar A, Mirzaei H. Anti-atherosclerotic effects of vitamins D and E in suppression of atherogenesis. J Cell Physiol. 2017;232:2968–76. https://doi.org/10.1002/jcp.25738.

119. Badimon L, Padró T, Vilahur G. Atherosclerosis, platelets and thrombosis in acute ischaemic heart disease. Eur Hear journal Acute Cardiovasc care. 2012;1:60–74. https://doi.org/10.1177/2048872612441582.

120. Gonzalez ER. Antiplatelet therapy in atherosclerotic cardiovascular disease. Clin Ther. 1998;20(Suppl B):B18–41.

121. Mekaj YH, Daci FT, Mekaj AY. New insights into the mechanisms of action of aspirin and its use in the prevention and treatment of arterial and venous thromboembolism. Ther Clin Risk Manag. 2015;11:1449–56. https://doi.org/10.2147/TCRM.S92222.

122. Phillips DR, Conley PB, Sinha U, Andre P. Therapeutic approaches in arterial thrombosis. J Thromb Haemost. 2005;3:1577–89. https://doi.org/10.1111/j.1538-7836.2005.01418.x.

123. Savi P, Herbert J-M. Clopidogrel and ticlopidine: P2Y12 adenosine diphosphate-receptor antagonists for the prevention of atherothrombosis. Semin Thromb Hemost. 2005;31:174–83. https://doi.org/10.1055/s-2005-869523.

124. Reaume KT, Regal RE, Dorsch MP. Indications for dual antiplatelet therapy with aspirin and clopidogrel: evidence-based recommendations for use. Ann Pharmacother. 2008;42:550–7. https://doi.org/10.1345/aph.1K433.

125. Giordano A, Musumeci G, D'Angelillo A, et al. Effects of glycoprotein iib/iiia antagonists: anti platelet aggregation and beyond. Curr Drug Metab. 2016;17:194–203.

126. Morrow DA, Braunwald E, Bonaca MP, et al. Vorapaxar in the secondary prevention of atherothrombotic events. N Engl J Med. 2012;366:1404–13. https://doi.org/10.1056/NEJMoa1200933.

127. Gresele P, Momi S. Inhibitors of the interaction between von Willebrand factor and platelet GPIb/IX/V. Handb Exp Pharmacol. 2012;287–309. https://doi.org/10.1007/978-3-642-29423-5_12.

128. Gresele P, Momi S. Pharmacologic profile and therapeutic potential of NCX 4016, a nitric oxide-releasing aspirin, for cardiovascular disorders. Cardiovasc Drug Rev. 2006;24:148–68. https://doi.org/10.1111/j.1527-3466.2006.00148.x.

129. Gayle RB, Maliszewski CR, Gimpel SD, et al. Inhibition of platelet function by recombinant soluble ecto-ADPase/CD39. J Clin Invest. 1998;101:1851–9. https://doi.org/10.1172/JCI1753.

130. Wiysonge CS, Volmink J, Opie LH. Beta-blockers and the treatment of hypertension: it is time to move on. Cardiovasc J Afr. 2007;18:351–2.

131. Maguire JJ, Davenport AP. Endothelin receptors and their antagonists. Semin Nephrol. 2015;35:125–36. https://doi.org/10.1016/j.semnephrol.2015.02.002.

132. Herman LL, Bhimji SS. Angiotensin Converting Enzyme Inhibitors (ACEI); 2018.

133. Laufs U, Gertz K, Huang P, et al. Atorvastatin upregulates type III nitric oxide synthase in thrombocytes, decreases platelet activation, and protects from cerebral ischemia in normocholesterolemic mice. Stroke. 2000;31:2442–9.

134. Ridker PM, Thuren T, Zalewski A, Libby P. Interleukin-1β inhibition and the prevention of recurrent cardiovascular events: rationale and design of the Canakinumab Anti-inflammatory Thrombosis Outcomes Study (CANTOS). Am Heart J. 2011;162:597–605. https://doi.org/10.1016/j.ahj.2011.06.012.

135. Ridker PM, Rifai N, Clearfield M, et al. Measurement of C-reactive protein for the targeting of statin therapy in the primary prevention of acute coronary events. N Engl J Med. 2001;344:1959–65. https://doi.org/10.1056/NEJM200106283442601.

136. Musial J, Undas A, Gajewski P, et al. Anti-inflammatory effects of simvastatin in subjects with hypercholesterolemia. Int J Cardiol. 2001;77:247–53.

137. Ridker PM. Inflammatory biomarkers, statins, and the risk of stroke: cracking a clinical conundrum. Circulation. 2002;105:2583–5.

138. Ridker PM, Rifai N, Pfeffer MA, et al. Long-term effects of pravastatin on plasma concentration of C-reactive protein. The Cholesterol and Recurrent Events (CARE) Investigators. Circulation. 1999;100:230–5.

139. Ridker PM, Cushman M, Stampfer MJ, et al. Plasma concentration of C-reactive protein and risk of developing peripheral vascular disease. Circulation. 1998;97:425–8.

140. Ridker PM, Cannon CP, Morrow D, et al. C-reactive protein levels and outcomes after statin therapy. N Engl J Med. 2005;352:20–8. https://doi.org/10.1056/NEJMoa042378.

141. Zhou Q, Liao JK. Pleiotropic effects of statins. - Basic research and clinical perspectives -. Circ J. 2010;74:818–26.

142. Scalia R, Stalker TJ. Microcirculation as a target for the anti-inflammatory properties of statins. Microcirculation. 2002;9:431–42. https://doi.org/10.1038/sj.mn.7800168.

143. Huang PL, Huang Z, Mashimo H, et al. Hypertension in mice lacking the gene for endothelial nitric oxide synthase. Nature. 1995;377:239–42. https://doi.org/10.1038/377239a0.

144. Radomski MW, Palmer RM, Moncada S. Endogenous nitric oxide inhibits human platelet adhesion to vascular endothelium. Lancet (London, England). 1987;2:1057–8.

145. Kubes P, Suzuki M, Granger DN. Nitric oxide: an endogenous modulator of leukocyte adhesion. Proc Natl Acad Sci. 1991;88:4651–5. https://doi.org/10.1073/pnas.88.11.4651.

146. Laufs U, La Fata V, Plutzky J, Liao JK. Upregulation of endothelial nitric oxide synthase by HMG CoA reductase inhibitors. Circulation. 1998;97:1129–35.

147. Laufs U, La Fata V, Liao JK. Inhibition of 3-Hydroxy-3-methylglutaryl (HMG)-CoA reductase blocks hypoxia-mediated down-regulation of endothelial nitric oxide synthase. J Biol Chem. 1997;272:31725–9. https://doi.org/10.1074/jbc.272.50.31725.

148. Wagner AH, Köhler T, Rückschloss U, et al. Improvement of nitric oxide-dependent vasodilatation by HMG-CoA reductase inhibitors through attenuation of endothelial superoxide anion formation. Arterioscler Thromb Vasc Biol. 2000;20:61–9.

149. Davignon J, Laaksonen R. Low-density lipoprotein-independent effects of statins. Curr Opin Lipidol. 1999;10:543–59.

150. Pruefer D, Scalia R, Lefer AM. Simvastatin inhibits leukocyte-endothelial cell interactions and protects against inflammatory processes in normocholesterolemic rats. Arterioscler Thromb Vasc Biol. 1999;19:2894–900.

151. Mueck AO, Seeger H, Wallwiener D. Further evidence for direct vascular actions of statins: effect on endothelial nitric oxide synthase and adhesion molecules. Exp Clin Endocrinol Diabetes. 2001;109:181–3. https://doi.org/10.1055/s-2001-14843.

152. Rezaie-Majd A, Prager GW, Bucek RA, et al. Simvastatin reduces the expression of adhesion molecules in circulating monocytes from hypercholesterolemic patients. Arterioscler Thromb Vasc Biol. 2003;23:397–403. https://doi.org/10.1161/01.ATV.0000059384.34874.F0.

153. Weitz-Schmidt G, Welzenbach K, Brinkmann V, et al. Statins selectively inhibit leukocyte function antigen-1 by binding to a novel regulatory integrin site. Nat Med. 2001;7:687–92. https://doi.org/10.1038/89058.

154. Peng H, Luo P, Li Y, et al. Simvastatin alleviates hyperpermeability of glomerular endothelial cells in early-stage diabetic nephropathy by inhibition of RhoA/ROCK1. PLoS ONE. 2013;8:e80009. https://doi.org/10.1371/journal.pone.0080009.

155. Huhle G, Abletshauser C, Mayer N, et al. Reduction of platelet activity markers in type II hypercholesterolemic patients by a HMG-CoA-reductase inhibitor. Thromb Res. 1999;95:229–34.

156. Hale LP, Craver KT, Berrier AM, et al. Combination of fosinopril and pravastatin decreases platelet response to thrombin receptor agonist in monkeys. Arterioscler Thromb Vasc Biol. 1998;18:1643–6.

157. Lacoste L, Lam JY, Hung J, et al. Hyperlipidemia and coronary disease. Correction of the increased thrombogenic potential with cholesterol reduction. Circulation. 1995;92:3172–7.

158. Park A, Barrera-Ramirez J, Ranasinghe I, et al. Use of statins to augment progenitor cell function in preclinical and clinical studies of regenerative therapy: a systematic review. Stem Cell Rev. 2016;12:327–39. https://doi.org/10.1007/s12015-016-9647-7.

159. Dimmeler S, Aicher A, Vasa M, et al. HMG-CoA reductase inhibitors (statins) increase endothelial progenitor cells via the PI 3-kinase/Akt pathway. J Clin Invest. 2001;108:391–7. https://doi.org/10.1172/JCI13152.

160. Landmesser U, Engberding N, Bahlmann FH, et al. Statin-induced improvement of endothelial progenitor cell mobilization, myocardial neovascularization, left ventricular function, and survival after experimental myocardial infarction requires endothelial nitric oxide synthase. Circulation. 2004;110:1933–9. https://doi.org/10.1161/01.CIR.0000143232.67642.7A.

161. Hristov M, Fach C, Becker C, et al. Reduced numbers of circulating endothelial progenitor cells in patients with coronary artery disease associated with long-term statin treatment. Atherosclerosis. 2007;192:413–20. https://doi.org/10.1016/j.atherosclerosis.2006.05.031.

162. Thompson PD, Buchner D, Pina IL, et al. Exercise and physical activity in the prevention and treatment of atherosclerotic cardiovascular disease: a statement from the Council on Clinical Cardiology (Subcommittee on Exercise, Rehabilitation, and Prevention) and the Council on Nutrition, Physical. Circulation. 2003;107:3109–16. https://doi.org/10.1161/01.CIR.0000075572.40158.77.

163. Leon AS, Franklin BA, Costa F, et al. Cardiac rehabilitation and secondary prevention of coronary heart disease: an American Heart Association scientific statement from the Council on Clinical Cardiology (Subcommittee on Exercise, Cardiac Rehabilitation, and Prevention) and the Council on Nut. Circulation. 2005;111:369–76. https://doi.org/10.1161/01.CIR.0000151788.08740.5C.

164. Taylor RS, Brown A, Ebrahim S, et al. Exercise-based rehabilitation for patients with coronary heart disease: systematic review and meta-analysis of randomized controlled trials. Am J Med. 2004;116:682–92. https://doi.org/10.1016/j.amjmed.2004.01.009.

165. Lawler PR, Filion KB, Eisenberg MJ. Efficacy of exercise-based cardiac rehabilitation post-myocardial infarction: a systematic review and meta-analysis of randomized controlled trials. Am Heart J. 2011;162:571–584.e2. https://doi.org/10.1016/j.ahj.2011.07.017.

166. Whelton SP, Chin A, Xin X, He J. Effect of aerobic exercise on blood pressure: a meta-analysis of randomized, controlled trials. Ann Intern Med. 2002;136:493–503.

167. Ross R, Dagnone D, Jones PJ, et al. Reduction in obesity and related comorbid conditions after diet-induced weight loss or exercise-induced weight loss in men. A randomized, controlled trial. Ann Intern Med. 2000;133:92–103.

168. Ross R, Janssen I, Dawson J, et al. Exercise-induced reduction in obesity and insulin resistance in women: a randomized controlled trial. Obes Res. 2004;12:789–98. https://doi.org/10.1038/oby.2004.95.

169. Irwin ML, Yasui Y, Ulrich CM, et al. Effect of exercise on total and intra-abdominal body fat in postmenopausal women: a randomized controlled trial. JAMA. 2003;289:323–30.

170. Kodama S, Tanaka S, Saito K, et al. Effect of aerobic exercise training on serum levels of high-density lipoprotein cholesterol: a meta-analysis. Arch Intern Med. 2007;167:999–1008. https://doi.org/10.1001/archinte.167.10.999.

171. Pearson MJ, Smart NA. Effect of exercise training on endothelial function in heart failure patients: a systematic review meta-analysis. Int J Cardiol. 2017;231:234–43. https://doi.org/10.1016/j.ijcard.2016.12.145.

172. Ashor AW, Lara J, Siervo M, et al. Exercise modalities and endothelial function: a systematic review and dose-response meta-analysis of randomized controlled trials. Sports Med. 2015;45:279–96. https://doi.org/10.1007/s40279-014-0272-9.

173. Laufs U, Werner N, Link A, et al. Physical training increases endothelial progenitor cells, inhibits neointima formation, and enhances angiogenesis. Circulation. 2004;109:220–6. https://doi.org/10.1161/01.CIR.0000109141.48980.37.

174. Rehman J, Li J, Parvathaneni L, et al. Exercise acutely increases circulating endothelial progenitor cells and monocyte-/macrophage-derived angiogenic cells. J Am Coll Cardiol. 2004;43:2314–8. https://doi.org/10.1016/j.jacc.2004.02.049.

175. De Biase C, De Rosa R, Luciano R, et al. Effects of physical activity on endothelial progenitor cells (EPCs). Front Physiol. 2013;4:414. https://doi.org/10.3389/fphys.2013.00414.

176. Kasapis C, Thompson PD. The effects of physical activity on serum C-reactive protein and inflammatory markers: a systematic review. J Am Coll Cardiol. 2005;45:1563–9. https://doi.org/10.1016/j.jacc.2004.12.077.

177. Woods JA, Wilund KR, Martin SA, Kistler BM. Exercise, inflammation and aging. Aging Dis. 2012;3:130–40.

178. Chen Y-W, Apostolakis S, Lip GYH. Exercise-induced changes in inflammatory processes: implications for thrombogenesis in cardiovascular disease. Ann Med. 2014;46:439–55. https://doi.org/10.3109/07853890.2014.927713.

179. Gomez-Cabrera M-C, Domenech E, Viña J. Moderate exercise is an antioxidant: upregulation of antioxidant genes by training. Free Radic Biol Med. 2008;44:126–31. https://doi.org/10.1016/j.freeradbiomed.2007.02.001.

180. de Sousa CV, Sales MM, Rosa TS, et al. The antioxidant effect of exercise: a systematic review and meta-analysis. Sport Med. 2017;47:277–93. https://doi.org/10.1007/s40279-016-0566-1.

181. Posthuma JJ, van der Meijden PEJ, Ten Cate H, Spronk HMH. Short- and Long-term exercise induced alterations in haemostasis: a review of the literature. Blood Rev. 2015;29:171–8. https://doi.org/10.1016/j.blre.2014.10.005.

182. Beiter T, Fragasso A, Hudemann J, et al. Neutrophils release extracellular DNA traps in response to exercise. J Appl Physiol. 2014;117:325–33. https://doi.org/10.1152/japplphysiol.00173.2014.

183. Beiter T, Hoene M, Prenzler F, et al. Exercise, skeletal muscle and inflammation: ARE-binding proteins as key regulators in inflammatory and adaptive networks. Exerc Immunol Rev. 2015;21:42–57.

184. Desai P, Williams AG, Prajapati P, Downey HF. Lymph flow in instrumented dogs varies with exercise intensity. Lymphat Res Biol. 2010;8:143–8. https://doi.org/10.1089/lrb.2009.0029.

185. Boulé NG, Haddad E, Kenny GP, et al. Effects of exercise on glycemic control and body mass in type 2 diabetes mellitus: a meta-analysis of controlled clinical trials. JAMA. 2001;286:1218–27.

186. Röhling M, Herder C, Roden M, et al. Effects of long-term exercise interventions on glycaemic control in type 1 and type 2 diabetes: a systematic review. Exp Clin Endocrinol Diabetes. 2016;124:487–94. https://doi.org/10.1055/s-0042-106293.

187. Blondell SJ, Hammersley-Mather R, Veerman JL. Does physical activity prevent cognitive decline and dementia?: a systematic review and meta-analysis of longitudinal studies. BMC Public Health. 2014;14:510. https://doi.org/10.1186/1471-2458-14-510.

188. Laver K, Dyer S, Whitehead C, et al. Interventions to delay functional decline in people with dementia: a systematic review of systematic reviews. BMJ Open. 2016;6:e010767. https://doi.org/10.1136/bmjopen-2015-010767.

189. Hernández SSS, Sandreschi PF, da Silva FC, et al. What are the benefits of exercise for Alzheimer's disease? A systematic review of the past 10 years. J Aging Phys Act. 2015;23:659–68. https://doi.org/10.1123/japa.2014-0180.

190. Pitkälä KH, Pöysti MM, Laakkonen M-L, et al. Effects of the finnish Alzheimer disease exercise trial (FINALEX): a randomized controlled trial. JAMA Intern Med. 2013;173:894–901. https://doi.org/10.1001/jamainternmed.2013.359.

191. Jick H, Zornberg GL, Jick SS, et al. Statins and the risk of dementia. Lancet (London, England). 2000;356:1627–31.

192. Chu C-S, Tseng P-T, Stubbs B, et al. Use of statins and the risk of dementia and mild cognitive impairment: a systematic review and meta-analysis. Sci Rep. 2018;8:5804. https://doi.org/10.1038/s41598-018-24248-8.

193. Zissimopoulos JM, Barthold D, Brinton RD, Joyce G. Sex and race differences in the association between statin use and the incidence of Alzheimer disease. JAMA Neurol. 2017;74:225–32. https://doi.org/10.1001/jamaneurol.2016.3783.

194. Koelwyn GJ, Quail DF, Zhang X, et al. Exercise-dependent regulation of the tumour microenvironment. Nat Rev Cancer. 2017;17:620–32. https://doi.org/10.1038/nrc.2017.78.

195. Demierre M-F, Higgins PDR, Gruber SB, et al. Statins and cancer prevention. Nat Rev Cancer. 2005;5:930–42. https://doi.org/10.1038/nrc1751.

196. Mei Z, Liang M, Li L, et al. Effects of statins on cancer mortality and progression: A systematic review and meta-analysis of 95 cohorts including 1,111,407 individuals. Int J Cancer. 2017;140:1068–81. https://doi.org/10.1002/ijc.30526.

197. Kyu HH, Bachman VF, Alexander LT, et al. Physical activity and risk of breast cancer, colon cancer, diabetes, ischemic heart disease, and ischemic stroke events: systematic review and dose-response meta-analysis for the Global Burden of Disease Study 2013. BMJ. 2016;354:i3857.

198. Al-Zahrani MS, Borawski EA, Bissada NF. Periodontitis and three health-enhancing behaviors: maintaining normal weight, engaging in recommended level of exercise, and consuming a high-quality diet. J Periodontol. 2005;76:1362–6. https://doi.org/10.1902/jop.2005.76.8.1362.

199. Estanislau IMG, Terceiro IRC, Lisboa MRP, et al. Pleiotropic effects of statins on the treatment of chronic periodontitis–a systematic review. Br J Clin Pharmacol. 2015;79:877–85. https://doi.org/10.1111/bcp.12564.

200. Hallsworth K, Fattakhova G, Hollingsworth KG, et al. Resistance exercise reduces liver fat and its mediators in non-alcoholic fatty liver disease independent of weight loss. Gut. 2011;60:1278–83. https://doi.org/10.1136/gut.2011.242073.

201. Hashida R, Kawaguchi T, Bekki M, et al. Aerobic vs. resistance exercise in non-alcoholic fatty liver disease: a systematic review. J Hepatol. 2017;66:142–52. https://doi.org/10.1016/j.jhep.2016.08.023.

202. Athyros VG, Alexandrides TK, Bilianou H, et al. The use of statins alone, or in combination with pioglitazone and other drugs, for the treatment of non-alcoholic fatty liver disease/non-alcoholic steatohepatitis and related cardiovascular risk. An expert panel statement. Metabolism. 2017;71:17–32. https://doi.org/10.1016/j.metabol.2017.02.014.

Chapter 6
New Ways to Target Vasa Vasorum for the Prevention and Treatment of Atherosclerosis

6.1 General

Based on the premise that vasa vasorum and their dysfunction are involved in the initiation and progression of atherosclerosis and are later implicated in plaque destabilization, one can understand why the current drug therapies are, for the most part, effective. As discussed in Chap. 5, anti-thrombotic drugs help prevent vasa vasorum obstruction, anti-hypertensive drugs help prevent vasa vasorum constriction, anti-inflammatory drugs reduce vasa vasorum leakiness, and lipid-lowering drugs have both an anti-inflammatory effect as well as prevent the deposition of cholesterol into vessel wall via leaky vasa vasorum. However, several new therapeutic opportunities focusing on preventing vasa vasorum dysfunction can be envisioned. This could be achieved by targeting newly recognized thrombotic components (e.g., NETs) as well as cell-specific and cell-state-specific signaling events that regulate endothelial cell differentiation, integrity, metabolism, or inflammatory or angiogenic responses (Fig. 6.1).

6.2 Preventing NET-Dependent Vasa Vasorum Obstruction

NETs can contribute to vessel occlusion including the microvasculature [1]. NETs provide a scaffold and stimulus for thrombus formation, stimulating immune cells to release pro-atherogenic cytokines [2, 3] and to promote clotting [4, 5]. Oxidized LDL [6], cholesterol crystals [7], and both type 1 and 2 diabetes [8–10] have been linked to NETosis. Therefore, as covered in Chap. 5, targeting NETosis with cholesterol-lowering, diabetic, and anti-inflammatory drugs such as statins or metformin reduces NET formation and thus likely reduces NET-induced

© Springer Nature Switzerland AG 2019
A. Haverich and E. C. Boyle, *Atherosclerosis Pathogenesis and Microvascular Dysfunction*, https://doi.org/10.1007/978-3-030-20245-3_6

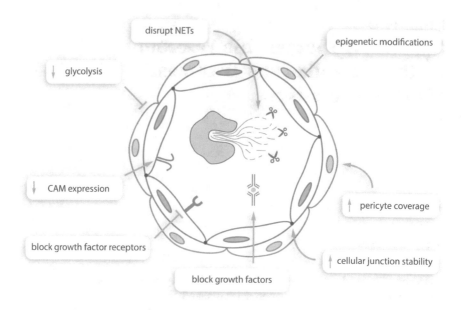

Fig. 6.1 Schematic of an arterial vasa vasorum and overview of therapeutic strategies to prevent vasa vasorum dysfunction

microthrombi [11, 12]. Several new strategies focused on NETosis are being explored. NETs contain extracellular chromatin with granular and cytoplasmic proteins [4, 13–16]. This offers another approach to treating vessel obstruction by transforming the DNA structure of NETs [17]. For example, DNase I can dissolve NETs [18] and DNase I treatment protects mice against NET-dependent deep vein thrombosis [19]. In rats with myocardial injury caused by NET-induced microthrombosis, treatment with DNase I plus recombinant tissue-type plasminogen activator reduces NET density, improves coronary microvasculature patency, limits infarct size, and attenuates long-term postinfarction left ventricular remodeling [20]. In humans, increased levels of circulating dsDNA, nucleosomes, and myeloperoxidase–DNA complexes are associated with severe coronary atherosclerosis, and could be targets for DNase therapy [21].

Chromatin decondensation is crucial to NET formation and is highly associated with histone citrullination [22]. NETs contain deiminated histones, and it was shown that peptidylarginine deiminase 4 (PAD4), which deiminates histones, is involved in NETosis [23, 24]. In ApoE$^{-/-}$ mice, PAD inhibition blocks NET formation and protects against atherosclerosis and NET-dependent arterial thrombosis [14]. Therefore, specific targeting of NETs is a promising future therapy in the prevention and treatment of vasa vasorum dysfunction and atherosclerosis.

6.3 Reducing Leakiness of Vasa Vasorum Neovessels

The barrier function of the endothelium is maintained by cellular junctions and can be affected by the extent of pericyte coverage. As mentioned in Chap. 4, leaky vasa vasorum have been implicated in all stages of atherosclerosis development from initiation, plaque growth, to thrombus formation. **Preserving integrity of the endothelium, especially in the vasa vasorum, is therefore another promising strategy for treating atherosclerosis.** Interesting targets to reestablish endothelial integrity are the main orchestrators of angiogenesis and vascular maturation such as VEGF and its receptors, matrix proteins, or the angiopoietin family.

VEGFs loosen endothelial junctions to allow angiogenic sprouting, which in parallel inherently causes vessel leakage. Several VEGF subtypes with high affinity for the VEGFR-2 receptor (i.e., VEGF-A and VEGF-F) are able to induce vascular hyperpermeability in a time-dependent and tissue-specific manner [25]. VEGF (preferably subtype-specific) inhibition could be a promising approach to reduce plaque vasa vasorum dysfunction, in addition to its anti-angiogenic properties. However, given the extensive physiologically important functions of VEGF, it may be preferable to interfere with signaling downstream of the VEGF pathway as identified by Laakkonen et al. [25], e.g., SNAI2, RCAN1, MYCN, and NR4A1.

Thrombospondin 1 is one of a family of secreted extracellular matrix proteins involved in angiogenesis and various other aspects of atherosclerotic pathophysiology [26]. One family member, thrombospondin type I domain 1 (THSD1), is involved in vascular integrity and plaque stability [27]. In human carotid endarterectomy specimens, THSD1 expression by endothelial cells was detected in advanced atherosclerotic lesions with intraplaque hemorrhage, but was absent in stable plaques. This implies that THSD1 is involved in neovascular bleeding. In vitro, pro-atherogenic factors (3% O_2 and TNFα) decreased THSD1 expression in human endothelial cells, whereas an anti-atherogenic factor (IL-10) had the opposite effect [27]. Therapeutic evaluation of mice with advanced atherosclerosis showed that THSD1 overexpression decreased plaque vulnerability by reducing vascular leakage in the lesions. This reduced macrophage accumulation and necrotic core size. Therefore, THSD1 looks to be an interesting drug target to treat microvascular pathologies in which endothelial barrier function is compromised.

Angiopoietin-2 (Ang-2) is a vascular growth factor that increases endothelial permeability and decreases pericyte recruitment. Conversely, Ang-1 has the opposite effect on the endothelium, promoting a mature, quiescent state and increasing the stability of endothelial junctions [28]. Moreover, it was shown that the balance between Ang-1 and -2 correlates with intraplaque microvessel density in human atherosclerotic plaques, in which the relative abundance of Ang-2 increases microvessel quantity [29]. Despite the beneficial effects of Ang-2 inhibition in several types of cancer [30, 31], a study examining the effects of Ang-2 inhibition in hypercholesterolemic mice found only a moderate decrease in early plaque development (fatty streak formation) but no effect on adventitial microvessel density or preexisting plaque size or composition [32]. This data demonstrates that inhibiting Ang-2 is not sufficient to affect preexisting atherosclerosis and additional factors need to be targeted as well.

Pericytes are contractile cells that wrap around endothelial cells that line arterioles, capillaries, venules, and vasa vasorum [33]. In response to angiogenic signals, pericytes detach and migrate away from the endothelium thereby contributing to leaky intercellular junctions. Therefore, pericytes play an important role in stabilizing the integrity of the microvasculature [34]. Sluimer and colleagues studied the ultrastructural integrity of vasa vasorum in human coronary arteries at autopsy [35]. They found that the endothelium of interplaque vasa vasorum was abnormal and demonstrated basal membrane detachment, open endothelial junctions, membrane blebs, intracytoplasmic vacuoles, and evidence of microvascular leakage. Interestingly, pericytes were conspicuously absent around interplaque vasa vasorum. Unfortunately, very little is known about the contribution of vasa vasorum-associated pericytes to plaque development. From other fields, we know that platelet-derived growth factor B (PDGF-B) plays a role in pericyte recruitment at the blood–brain barrier [36]. Mice deficient in the PDGF-B retention motif (PDGF-B ret/ret) have diminished pericyte coverage leading to permeability of the blood–brain barrier [37]. Moreover, the aforementioned VEGF inhibitor bevacizumab was shown to reduce vascular leakage by restoring pericyte function through induction of PDGF-B expression in vivo in a hindlimb ischemia mouse model [38]. Interestingly, in light of cardiovascular event prevention, the extensively used HMGCoA-reductase inhibitors ("statins") have been shown to increase apoptotic cell death of pericytes both in vitro and in vivo, possibly counteracting their anti-atherogenic features by destabilizing plaques [39].

In summary, there are several pathways and mechanisms involved in endothelial barrier destabilization, and thus multiple plausible targets to prevent this. VEGF subtypes appear especially interesting as these keep emerging as important players in different pathways. Unfortunately, VEGFs are involved in important physiological processes and therefore perhaps it is not surprising that multiple trials with VEGF inhibiting compounds also show harmful effects (e.g., hypertension, arterial thromboembolic events, and cardiotoxicity). For example, despite some promising results with the VEGF-A inhibitor bevacizumab on tumor angiogenesis, some serious adverse cardiovascular events (angina pectoris, arterial thrombosis, cerebral or myocardial ischemia, and infarction) have been reported [40]. This is of particular relevance for its potential use as atherosclerosis therapy, as a history of this disease greatly enhances the risk of cardiovascular events. The so-called "Janus" face of VEGF is explained by its positive effect on maintenance and regeneration of arterial endothelium, as opposed to its destabilizing effect on microvascular endothelium. Similar concerns for the increased risk of stroke have been described for the intraocular use of the VEGF-A inhibitor ranibizumab [41], suggesting that VEGF inhibition in general should be used with caution.

6.4 Inhibiting Maladaptive Angiogenesis

Much of what we know about anti-angiogenic therapies has been drawn from the field of cancer where they have been used to fight tumor cell growth [42–44]. In experimental atherosclerosis in animal models, the use of angiogenic inhibitors has shown that pathogenic expansion of vasa vasorum can be reduced. Thalidomide, a drug originally used as a sedative, has anti-inflammatory, anti-tumorigenic, and anti-angiogenic properties as it both inhibits growth factor production and leads to depletion of growth factor receptors [42, 45]. Thalidomide treatment of early atherosclerosis in hypercholesteremic pigs diminishes coronary vasa vasorum neovascularization, local tumor necrosis factor α (TNFα) production, and inhibits neointima formation [46]. Furthermore, in hypercholesteremic ApoE-deficient mice, thalidomide reduces plaque growth as well as vasa vasorum neovascularization [47]. Angiostatin is a proteolytic fragment of plasminogen that has a potent antagonistic effect on angiogenesis. Through its binding to ATP synthase on the endothelial cell surface, angiostatin leads to downregulation of cell migration and proliferation [48]. Angiostatin treatment of cholesterol-fed ApoE-deficient mice suppresses VEGF levels and vessel sprouting in the intima, thereby reducing vasa vasorum density [49]. Similarly, treatment of atherosclerosis-prone mice with the anti-angiogenic drugs endostatin or TNP-470 also inhibits endothelial cell proliferation and migration, limits plaque growth, and reduces intimal neovascularization by at least 70% [50]. The angiogenesis inhibitor rPAI-1₂₃ affects fibroblast growth factor (FGF)-stimulated endothelial cell migration, tube formation, and proliferation [51, 52]. When atherosclerosis-prone mice are treated with rPAI-1₂₃, vasa vasorum density, plaque area, and plaque cholesterol are all reduced [51].

In humans, angiogenesis inhibitors have been extensively studied in the treatment of cancer. Thalidomide, for example, has been used to treat multiple myeloma and other types of cancer that express angiogenic cytokines [53, 54]. However, the use of such drugs for atherosclerosis is still at an early stage. Thalidomide has been investigated in patients with chronic heart failure [55]. Those with cardiovascular artery disease demonstrated only a moderate increase in left ventricular function and more adverse events occurred compared to patients with other etiologies. From cancer studies, it is also well established that anti-angiogenic therapies often have transient effects because there are multiple compensatory mechanisms that take over [56]. In vitro overexpression of endogenous angiogenesis inhibitors in tumor cells initially leads to suppression of angiogenesis. However, all tumors ultimately escaped inhibition by upregulating pro-angiogenic factors, even when multiple inhibitors were expressed in combination. Therefore, more research is needed into the mechanisms of escape or evasion from angiogenesis inhibition. **For the long-term treatment of atherosclerosis, a future strategy could be the combination of anti-angiogenic with anti-inflammatory treatment regimes.**

6.5   Possibilities of Nanomedicine to Control Maladaptive Inflammation and Angiogenesis

One potential problem with many of the aforementioned treatments is that they act not only locally but also systemically. A clever tactic is the use of **nanoscale particles as carriers to deliver therapeutic agents to a desired diseased site** [57]. These particles can be designed in various sizes, shapes, and with different surface chemistries to affect their localization and behavior in vivo [58–61]. Therefore, nanoparticles can improve a drug's therapeutic index, increasing its on-target efficacy and at the same time reducing any detrimental off-target effects or toxicity. Drug delivery systems include micelles, liposomes, polymeric nanoparticles, dendrimers, carbon nanotubes, and crystalline metals [62].

So far, nanomedicine to target angiogenesis has mainly been studied for cancer therapy. TNP-70 is the water soluble form of fumagillin, a mycotoxin of *Aspergillus fumigatus* and potent anti-angiogenic compound. Unfortunately, TNP-470 causes significant side effects, most commonly neurotoxicity, at dosages required for therapeutic effects. Site-directed delivery of this drug significantly reduces the dose needed and therefore would be highly desirable. Recently, APRPG (Ala-Pro-Arg-Pro-Gly) peptide-modified poly (ethylene glycol)-poly (lactic acid) (PEG-PLA) nanoparticles (NP-APRPG) encapsulating TNP-470 (TNP-470-NP-APRPG) were designed and tested in a cancer model [63]. In this configuration, maleimide-PEG-PLA and mPEG-PLA served as carrier materials, an APRPG peptide specifically targeted integrins highly expressed in neovessels, PEG prolonged circulation in vivo, and PLA was used to load the anti-angiogenesis drug TNP-470. Tested in an animal model of ovarian cancer, TNP-470-NP-APRPG significantly reduced angiogenesis and retarded tumor growth. A similar approach was used to target maladaptive angiogenesis in relation to atherosclerosis using integrin-targeted fumagillin nanoparticles. In hyperlipidemic rabbits, integrin-targeted fumagillin nanoparticles significantly reduced aortic neovessel formation, especially in combination with statin therapy [64, 65]. In the future, APRPG peptide-modified nanoparticles hold a lot of promise to specifically target vasa vasorum dysfunction.

Therapeutic nanoparticles can also be specifically targeted to inflammatory cells which preferentially home to the inflamed endothelium of vasa vasorum neovessels. Since macrophages naturally migrate to sites of atherosclerosis, nanoparticle-laden macrophages can act like Trojan horses delivering anti-atherogenic drugs to the vasa vasorum. For example, poly(lactic-co-glycolic acid) (PLGA) nanoparticles are known to target inflammatory cells (mainly monocytes) when administered intravenously [66, 67]. By incorporating a statin into PLGA nanoparticles, plaque destabilization and rupture were prevented when administered intravenously into atherosclerotic mice [66]. Another approach is to use macrophage-targeted nanoparticles to shift them into a less inflammatory state. For example, peroxisome proliferator-activated receptor-γ induces a polarity shift in monocytes/macrophages toward a less inflammatory phenotype and thereby has the potential to prevent atherosclerotic plaque ruptures. By incorporating the peroxisome proliferator-activated receptor-γ agonist pioglitazone into PLGA nanoparticles, plaque destabilization and rupture could be prevented when administered intravenously into atherosclerotic mice [67]. Beldman and colleagues used hyaluronan nanoparticles that selectively target plaque-associated macrophages, dampening inflammation and improving plaque stability in atherosclerotic mice [68]. And since inflammation and angiogenesis are codependent, a decrease in plaque inflammation likely also affects plaque angiogenesis.

The endothelium of vasa vasorum can also be targeted by nanoparticle-based therapies. As previously mentioned, endothelial cells of the vasa vasorum express especially high amounts of cell adhesion molecules compared to the parent vessel. Sager and colleagues were able to successfully silence expression of five different endothelial cell adhesion molecules (ICAMs, VCAMs, selectins) using siRNA-loaded endothelial-avid nanoparticles [69]. In ApoE$^{-/-}$ mice with accelerated atherosclerosis after MI, neutrophil and monocyte recruitment into atherosclerotic lesions was significantly decreased. Reduced inflammation of the infarcted myocardium and improved recovery after ischemia in mice were the result.

In humans, the use of nanoparticle-based therapies is still in its infancy [70]. An innovative option is using nanoparticles that combine molecular imaging and drug delivery [61]. This way the disease burden can be determined, the drug can be delivered at a lower concentration, and the local response can be assessed. The recent design and screening of an extensive library of nanoparticles based on endogenous high-density lipoprotein found a number of promising candidates that could be used for preferential delivery of therapeutic compounds to pathological macrophages in atherosclerosis [71]. Overall, the biocompatibility, site-specific targeting, drug-loading capacity, and in vivo persistence are necessary prerequisites for nanoparticle efficacy and their potential clinical application.

6.6   Targeting Cellular Metabolism to Maintain Vasa Vasorum Quiescence

Mature, quiescent endothelial cells lining the blood, and lymphatic vasculature maintain redox homeostasis and have optimized cellular repair mechanisms. Triggered by ischemia, injury, or inflammation, endothelial cells can rapidly switch from a quiescent to an angiogenic state. This switch requires a change in endothelial cell metabolism since angiogenesis is an energy-demanding process. To support sprouting, migration, and proliferation, endothelial cells rely heavily on glycolysis for ATP generation [72]. **Targeting this cellular metabolic pathway is a relatively new therapeutic strategy to limit pathological angiogenesis** [73–78]. 6-phosphofructo-2-kinase/fructose-2,6-biphosphatase 3 (PFKFB3) is a key glycolytic enzyme and is thus an attractive therapeutic target. PFKFB3 inhibitors have been shown to maintain endothelial cells in a quiescent state, reducing injury- and inflammation-induced pathological angiogenesis in vivo [78, 79].

Anti-angiogenic targeting of endothelial cell metabolism has been primarily investigated for cancer but has also garnered interest in the treatment of other diseases characterized by increased angiogenesis (e.g., macular degeneration, inflammatory bowel disease, and skin psoriasis) [79]. By shifting endothelial cells into a more quiescent state, proliferation is slowed, cellular junctions are stabilized, and expression of cellular adhesion molecules is reduced. Given that the pathological expansion and fragility of vasa vasorum neovessels likely contributes to atherosclerosis disease initiation and progression, inhibition of specific metabolic pathways in endothelial cells could be an attractive treatment strategy for atherosclerosis.

In cancer models, inhibition of PFKFB3 has been shown to impair nuclear factor kappa B (NF-κB) transcriptional activity in endothelial cells by targeting the phosphorylation of p65 and IκBα. A reduction in NF-κB activity subsequently results in less expression of cell adhesion molecules (CAMs) [80]. Compared to their parent vessels, vasa vasorum endothelial cells express higher levels of CAMs such as VCAM-1, ICAM-1, and E-selectin [81–83]. As vasa vasorum play an important role in the recruitment of inflammatory cells into atherosclerotic plaques, specific reduction of CAMs by a PFKFB3 inhibitor could influence plaque initiation and progression.

Quiescent endothelial layers are more stable and, in the case of microvasculature, are supported by pericyte coverage. Accordingly, **maintaining cells in a quiescent state could be used to stabilize the endothelial barrier of vasa vasorum and thereby controlling the initiation and progression of atherosclerosis.** Cancer model studies have shown that PFKFB3 inhibitors decrease pericyte glycolysis, consequently promoting pericyte quiescence and cell adhesiveness [80]. Tighter pericyte coverage of the microvasculature endothelium supports maturation and normalization of the tumor vasculature, preventing endothelial barrier leakiness. Similarly, targeting pericyte cell metabolism during the course of atherosclerosis could be beneficial in stabilizing vasa vasorum integrity [73, 84, 85].

Thus far, all experimentally tested glycolysis inhibitors have only partially and transiently inhibited glycolysis. This incomplete inhibition is likely advantageous because to maintain cell homeostasis, some glycolysis flux is required to avoid detrimental systemic side effects on glycolysis-dependent healthy tissues [79, 86]. In the case of using glycolysis inhibitors for atherosclerosis, one might hypothesize that a complete block of vasa vasorum neoangiogenesis could worsen vascular wall hypoxia thereby exacerbating plaque development. Thus, incomplete or partial inhibition of glycolysis may actually be ideal.

In an effort to study the metabolic characteristics of vasa vasorum endothelial cells associated with pulmonary hypertension, vasa vasorum endothelial cells were isolated from the pulmonary artery of chronically hypoxic, hypertensive calves [87, 88]. Glycolysis and oxidative phosphorylation were both highly upregulated and shown to be important for the angiogenic responses of vasa vasorum endothelial cells [87]. These findings suggest that metabolic pathways could be targeted to treat pathological microvascular remodeling during pulmonary hypertension. Future metabolic characterization vasa vasorum endothelial cells isolated from different vascular beds during diseased and non-diseased states could help to identify new therapeutic opportunities to target atherosclerotic neovessel metabolism.

6.7 Epigenetic Strategies to Target Microvascular Dysfunction

In response to environmental stimuli, epigenetic modifications such as DNA methylation and histone posttranslational modifications can modulate gene expression by changing the binding of specific transcription factors. **Epigenomic mapping has revealed several cell- and disease-stage-specific epigenetic changes that are associated with atherosclerosis** [89, 90]. We will highlight two examples of how atherogenic inflammatory factors affect the epigenetic machinery and how these pathways could be harnessed to render vasa vasorum endothelial cells less susceptible to inflammatory triggers.

OxLDL is a potent trigger of endothelial dysfunction. Upon exposure to oxLDL, endothelial cells upregulate expression of DNA methyltransferase (DNMT)1 which in turn methylates the promoter encoding the anti-inflammatory transcription factor Krüppel-like factor 2 (KLF2). Methylation of this promoter results in repression of KLF2 expression and consequent increased inflammation. The effect of oxLDL on KLF2 can be prevented through inhibition of DNMT1 by 5-aza-2′-deoxycytidine (5-AZA) [91] (Fig. 6.2). In atherosclerosis mouse models, 5-AZA significantly reduced plaque burden and the amount of macrophages within plaques [92, 93]. Therefore, reducing the endothelium's epigenetic response to oxLDL could slow disease progression by preventing inflammatory and angiogenic signaling.

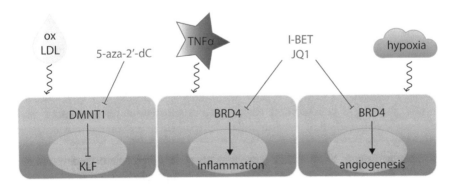

Fig. 6.2 Pharmacological inhibition of epigenetic modifications to dampen the response of the vasa vasorum endothelium to inflammatory stimuli. oxLDL, oxidized low-density lipoprotein; DMNT1, DNA methyltransferase 1; KLF2, Krüppel-like factor 2; BRD4, bromodomain-containing protein 4; 5-aza-2′-dC, 5-aza-2′-deoxycytidine. Reproduced from [73]

Inflammatory cytokines also induce epigenetic changes in endothelial cells which further drive inflammatory processes [89]. When endothelial cells are exposed to tumor necrosis factor α (TNFα), the transcription factor NF-κB interacts with chromatin regulators and the epigenetic reader bromodomain-containing protein 4 (BRD4) which are all then directed to enhancer regions. Through NF-kB-dependent redistribution of BRD4, super-enhancers are established allowing immediate transcriptional activation of pro-inflammatory genes. By inhibiting BRD4 in endothelial cells, the expression of pro-inflammatory cytokines and cell adhesion molecules is reduced. In a mouse model of atherosclerosis, BRD4 inhibition attenuates plaque burden and leukocyte extravasation into plaques. Moreover, bromodomain and extra terminal domain (BET) protein inhibitors, e.g., I-BET and JQ1, have also shown promise in reducing inflammation in preclinical models of rheumatoid arthritis, psoriasis, and sepsis [94]. With regard to atherosclerosis, **suppression of epigenetic modifications in vasa vasorum endothelial cells could render these cells less sensitive to inflammatory triggers** (e.g., oxLDL and TNFα) and thereby prevent inflammation-induced microvascular dysfunction (Fig. 6.2).

From the cancer field, we also know that endothelial cells undergo epigenetic changes in response to hypoxia. BET inhibitors dampen the endothelial cell response to hypoxia thereby reducing hypoxia-induced angiogenesis [95]. Whether BET inhibitors could modulate the response of vasa vasorum to hypoxic conditions is currently not known but would be an interesting avenue of research. In addition, determining the specific epigenetic modifications that occur in vasa vasorum endothelial cells under hypoxic and inflammatory conditions would help identify the best target molecules for therapeutic intervention. Similarly, specific targeting of epigenetic regulators of the neovasculature would allow site-specific targeting to maintain the vasa vasorum endothelial cells in a quiescent mature state.

6.8   Tackling Vasa Vasorum Dysfunction with MicroRNAs

MicroRNAs (miRNAs) are small noncoding RNAs that can target multiple genes and typically inhibit their expression. Many miRNAs are differentially expressed in a tissue-, cell type-, or disease state-specific manner making them attractive targets for precision therapy approaches targeting a specific cell type during a certain pathologic condition. **Altered miRNA expression is associated with atherosclerosis [96] and several miRNAs and their associated target genes can affect vascular remodeling.** Accordingly, miRNAs have become attractive therapeutic targets to modulate genes involved in atherosclerosis development [74, 97, 98]. However, the use of miRNAs is complicated by the fact that each miRNA is capable of affecting various, often unrelated genes [99]. Moreover, depending on the cell type, activation and/or differentiation state, and microenvironment, a given miRNA can have different effects. For example, upregulation of miR-126 is generally thought to have atheroprotective effects as it dampens inflammation-associated genes and inhibits angiogenesis in mature endothelial cells [100]. However, under hypoxic conditions, or in the case of vessel wall injury, miR-126 can stimulate the formation of neovessels, thereby assuming a pro-angiogenic function [101–103]. Because of hypoxic conditions, upregulation of miR-126 in vasa vasorum endothelial cells may have adverse effects resulting in a localized proliferation of unstable neovessels. MiR-221 and its paralogue miR-222 also have potentially conflicting effects on the endothelium [104]. While expression of miR-221/222 supports endothelial quiescence, they also downregulate endothelial nitric oxide synthase [105], resulting in possible endothelial dysfunction caused by oxidative stress and inflammation. Moreover, miR-221/222 are also expressed by vascular smooth muscle cells where they stimulate proliferation thereby accelerating neointima formation [106] which could then contribute to plaque progression.

Future research must clarify the role individual miRNAs play in the development and progression of atherosclerosis. Identifying the cell- and environment-specific signaling pathways and understanding the molecular and cellular pathways affected by each miRNA will be of utmost importance. Together with the feasibility of miRNA-inhibiting approaches in humans [107], the suitability of employing miRNAs to target vasa vasorum dysfunction holds much promise.

6.9   Drugging the Microbiome

As mentioned in Chap. 5, the intestinal microbiota indirectly affects thrombotic potential in vivo through TLR2-dependent regulation of endothelial vWF synthesis in the liver endothelium [108]. Determining whether specific members of the microbiota are responsible for TLR2-triggered vWF expression will be important for identifying druggable targets to combat thrombosis involved in atherosclerosis. In addition, these findings raise the possibility that infections (e.g., *Salmonella typhimurium*) or conditions (e.g., celiac disease) that disrupt the gut–vascular barrier [109] could increase levels of bacterial TLR ligands in portal circulation, thereby amplifying vWF synthesis and promoting thrombosis. **The recent discovery and appreciation of the importance of the gut–vascular barrier in the regulation of the gut–liver axis and hemostatic balance will open the doors to novel drug discoveries.**

In the intestine, the dietary nutrients phosphatidylcholine, choline, and carnitine are converted to trimethylamine (TMA) by the microbiota and then TMA is oxidized in the liver to TMAO. The diet- and microbiota-dependent metabolite TMAO is a newly identified risk factor for atherosclerosis and has been shown to directly stimulate platelet aggregation. The use of antiplatelet drugs in the treatment of cardiovascular disease is widespread however this approach always runs the risk of patients bleeding. This risk can be circumvented by targeting the specific microbial pathways which precipitate platelet aggregation. For example, drugging the microbial TMAO pathway has been successful in preventing thrombosis and attenuating atherosclerosis development in preclinical models. Treatment of mice with a nonlethal small molecule inhibitor of TMA lyase reduced circulating TMAO levels and abrogated choline diet-induced atherosclerosis development [110]. Further efforts by the same group discovered an even more potent and irreversible inhibitor of microbial TMA lyase. In animal models, a single oral dose of this next-generation TMA lyase inhibitor significantly reduced plasma TMAO levels for up to 3 days and prevented diet-induced platelet activation and thrombus formation [111]. Whether there are more microbe-derived metabolites capable of exacerbating or ameliorating atherosclerosis development is an important question for future research.

6.10 Conclusions and Future Perspectives

Robust scientific evidence documents a clear connection between dysfunctional vasa vasorum and all stages of atherosclerosis development—from vasa vasorum obstruction, malperfusion, or angiogenic expansion to atherosclerotic plaque growth and progression toward an inflammatory, unstable plaque phenotype. This leads to rupture and related clinical events. In physiological conditions, vasa vasorum enable the access of oxygen and nutrients to the vessel wall. However, when expanding due to pathological stimuli, vasa vasorum set the milieu for plaque growth and function as carriers of cholesterol, inflammatory cells, erythrocytes, provisional extracellular matrix, or other atherogenic molecules into the growing plaque. Conversely, prevention of new vasa vasorum growth or stabilization of existing physiological vasa vasorum is followed by a reduction in plaque growth and increased plaque stability. In spite of these clear relationships, the precise mechanisms regulating pathological vasa vasorum expansion are unknown. **The interplay between the multifactorial events determines the role of vasa vasorum in plaque growth, progression, and rupture.** So far, many therapeutic strategies to target the microvasculature have come from cancer research, and the focus is often on endothelial cells. While the association between vasa vasorum dysfunction and atherosclerosis is substantial, future therapeutic approaches specifically targeting the microvasculature in developing plaques will have to be established and evaluated. In particular, advances in the understanding of the metabolic and epigenetic players involved in the regulation of disease-specific functions of endothelial cells will enable the identification and development of new treatment modalities to treat atherosclerosis, permitting a precise and safe targeting of vasa vasorum.

References

1. Jiménez-Alcázar M, Napirei M, Panda R, et al. Impaired DNase1-mediated degradation of neutrophil extracellular traps is associated with acute thrombotic microangiopathies. J Thromb Haemost. 2015;13:732–42. https://doi.org/10.1111/jth.12796.

2. Goossens P, Gijbels MJJ, Zernecke A, et al. Myeloid type I interferon signaling promotes atherosclerosis by stimulating macrophage recruitment to lesions. Cell Metab. 2010;12:142–53. https://doi.org/10.1016/j.cmet.2010.06.008.

3. Li J, Fu Q, Cui H, et al. Interferon-α priming promotes lipid uptake and macrophage-derived foam cell formation: a novel link between interferon-α and atherosclerosis in lupus. Arthritis Rheum. 2011;63:492–502. https://doi.org/10.1002/art.30165.

4. Fuchs TA, Brill A, Duerschmied D, et al. Extracellular DNA traps promote thrombosis. Proc Natl Acad Sci USA. 2010;107:15880–5. https://doi.org/10.1073/pnas.1005743107.

5. Fuchs TA, Brill A, Wagner DD. Neutrophil extracellular trap (NET) impact on deep vein thrombosis. Arterioscler Thromb Vasc Biol. 2012;32:1777–83. https://doi.org/10.1161/ATVBAHA.111.242859.

6. Awasthi D, Nagarkoti S, Kumar A, et al. Oxidized LDL induced extracellular trap formation in human neutrophils via TLR-PKC-IRAK-MAPK and NADPH-oxidase activation. Free Radic Biol Med. 2016;93:190–203. https://doi.org/10.1016/j.freeradbiomed.2016.01.004.

7. Warnatsch A, Ioannou M, Wang Q, Papayannopoulos V. Neutrophil extracellular traps license macrophages for cytokine production in atherosclerosis. Science. 2015;349:316–320. https://doi.org/10.1126/science.aaa8064.

8. Wang Y, Xiao Y, Zhong L, et al. Increased neutrophil elastase and proteinase 3 and augmented NETosis are closely associated with β-cell autoimmunity in patients with type 1 diabetes. Diabetes. 2014;63:4239–48. https://doi.org/10.2337/db14-0480.

9. Menegazzo L, Ciciliot S, Poncina N, et al. NETosis is induced by high glucose and associated with type 2 diabetes. Acta Diabetol. 2015;52:497–503. https://doi.org/10.1007/s00592-014-0676-x.

10. Fadini GP, Menegazzo L, Rigato M, et al. NETosis delays diabetic wound healing in mice and humans. Diabetes. 2016;65:1061–71. https://doi.org/10.2337/db15-0863.

11. Menegazzo L, Scattolini V, Cappellari R, et al. The antidiabetic drug metformin blunts NETosis in vitro and reduces circulating NETosis biomarkers in vivo. Acta Diabetol. 2018;55:593–601. https://doi.org/10.1007/s00592-018-1129-8.

12. Al-Ghoul WM, Kim MS, Fazal N, et al. Evidence for simvastatin anti-inflammatory actions based on quantitative analyses of NETosis and other inflammation/oxidation markers. Results Immunol. 2014;4:14–22. https://doi.org/10.1016/j.rinim.2014.03.001.

13. Sørensen OE, Borregaard N. Neutrophil extracellular traps—the dark side of neutrophils. J Clin Invest. 2016;126:1612–20. https://doi.org/10.1172/JCI84538.

14. Knight JS, Luo W, O'Dell AA, et al. Peptidylarginine deiminase inhibition reduces vascular damage and modulates innate immune responses in murine models of atherosclerosis. Circ Res. 2014;114:947–56. https://doi.org/10.1161/CIRCRESAHA.114.303312.

15. Brinkmann V, Reichard U, Goosmann C, et al. Neutrophil extracellular traps kill bacteria. Science. 2004;303:1532–5. https://doi.org/10.1126/science.1092385.

16. Brinkmann V, Zychlinsky A. Neutrophil extracellular traps: is immunity the second function of chromatin? J Cell Biol. 2012;198:773–83. https://doi.org/10.1083/jcb.201203170.

17. Frese S, Diamond B. Structural modification of DNA—a therapeutic option in SLE? Nat Rev Rheumatol. 2011;7:733–8. https://doi.org/10.1038/nrrheum.2011.153.

18. Macanovic M, Sinicropi D, Shak S, et al. The treatment of systemic lupus erythematosus (SLE) in NZB/W F1 hybrid mice; studies with recombinant murine DNase and with dexamethasone. Clin Exp Immunol. 1996;106:243–52.

19. Brill A, Fuchs TA, Savchenko AS, et al. Neutrophil extracellular traps promote deep vein thrombosis in mice. J Thromb Haemost. 2012;10:136–44. https://doi. org/10.1111/j.1538-7836.2011.04544.x.
20. Ge L, Zhou X, Ji W-J, et al. Neutrophil extracellular traps in ischemia-reperfusion injury-induced myocardial no-reflow: therapeutic potential of DNase-based reperfusion strategy. Am J Physiol Heart Circ Physiol. 2015;308:H500–9. https://doi.org/10.1152/ ajpheart.00381.2014.
21. Borissoff JI, Joosen IA, Versteylen MO, et al. Elevated levels of circulating DNA and chromatin are independently associated with severe coronary atherosclerosis and a prothrombotic state. Arterioscler Thromb Vasc Biol. 2013;33:2032–40. https://doi. org/10.1161/ATVBAHA.113.301627.
22. Döring Y, Soehnlein O, Weber C. Neutrophil extracellular traps in atherosclerosis and atherothrombosis. Circ Res. 2017;120:736–43. https://doi.org/10.1161/ CIRCRESAHA.116.309692.
23. Rohrbach AS, Slade DJ, Thompson PR, Mowen KA. Activation of PAD4 in NET formation. Front Immunol. 2012;3:360. https://doi.org/10.3389/fimmu.2012.00360.
24. Leshner M, Wang S, Lewis C, et al. PAD4 mediated histone hypercitrullination induces heterochromatin decondensation and chromatin unfolding to form neutrophil extracellular trap-like structures. Front Immunol. 2012;3:307. https://doi.org/10.3389/ fimmu.2012.00307.
25. Laakkonen JP, Lappalainen JP, Theelen TL, et al. Differential regulation of angiogenic cellular processes and claudin-5 by histamine and VEGF via PI3 K-signaling, transcription factor SNAI2 and interleukin-8. Angiogenesis. 2017;20:109–24. https://doi.org/10.1007/ s10456-016-9532-7.
26. Stenina-Adognravi O. Thrombospondins. Curr Opin Lipidol. 2013;24:401–9. https://doi. org/10.1097/MOL.0b013e3283642912.
27. Haasdijk RA, Den Dekker WK, Cheng C, et al. THSD1 preserves vascular integrity and protects against intraplaque haemorrhaging in ApoE$^{-/-}$ mice. Cardiovasc Res. 2016;110:129–39. https://doi.org/10.1093/cvr/cvw015.
28. Thurston G, Suri C, Smith K, et al. Leakage-resistant blood vessels in mice transgenically overexpressing angiopoietin-1. Science. 1999;286:2511–4.
29. Post S, Peeters W, Busser E, et al. Balance between angiopoietin-1 and angiopoietin-2 is in favor of angiopoietin-2 in atherosclerotic plaques with high microvessel density. J Vasc Res. 2008;45:244–50. https://doi.org/10.1159/000112939.
30. Holopainen T, Saharinen P, D'Amico G, et al. Effects of angiopoietin-2-blocking antibody on endothelial cell-cell junctions and lung metastasis. J Natl Cancer Inst. 2012;104:461–75. https://doi.org/10.1093/jnci/djs009.
31. Leow CC, Coffman K, Inigo I, et al. MEDI3617, a human anti-angiopoietin 2 monoclonal antibody, inhibits angiogenesis and tumor growth in human tumor xenograft models. Int J Oncol. 2012;40:1321–30. https://doi.org/10.3892/ijo.2012.1366.
32. Theelen TL, Lappalainen JP, Sluimer JC, et al. Angiopoietin-2 blocking antibodies reduce early atherosclerotic plaque development in mice. Atherosclerosis. 2015;241:297–304. https://doi.org/10.1016/j.atherosclerosis.2015.05.018.
33. Attwell D, Mishra A, Hall CN, et al. What is a pericyte? J Cereb Blood Flow Metab. 2016;36:451–5. https://doi.org/10.1177/0271678X15610340.
34. Schrimpf C, Teebken OE, Wilhelmi M, Duffield JS. The role of pericyte detachment in vascular rarefaction. J Vasc Res. 2014;51:247–58. https://doi.org/10.1159/000365149.
35. Sluimer JC, Kolodgie FD, Bijnens APJJ, et al. Thin-walled microvessels in human coronary atherosclerotic plaques show incomplete endothelial junctions. J Am Coll Cardiol. 2009;53:1517–27. https://doi.org/10.1016/j.jacc.2008.12.056.
36. Lindblom P, Gerhardt H, Liebner S, et al. Endothelial PDGF-B retention is required for proper investment of pericytes in the microvessel wall. Genes Dev. 2003;17:1835–40. https://doi.org/10.1101/gad.266803.

37. Armulik A, Genové G, Mäe M, et al. Pericytes regulate the blood-brain barrier. Nature. 2010;468:557–61. https://doi.org/10.1038/nature09522.

38. Xiao L, Yan K, Yang Y, et al. Anti-vascular endothelial growth factor treatment induces blood flow recovery through vascular remodeling in high-fat diet induced diabetic mice. Microvasc Res. 2016;105:70–6. https://doi.org/10.1016/j.mvr.2016.01.005.

39. Bababeygy SR, Polevaya N V, Youssef S, et al. HMG-CoA reductase inhibition causes increased necrosis and apoptosis in an in vivo mouse glioblastoma multiforme model. Anticancer Res. 2009;29:4901–4908.

40. Scappaticci FA, Skillings JR, Holden SN, et al. Arterial thromboembolic events in patients with metastatic carcinoma treated with chemotherapy and bevacizumab. JNCI J Natl Cancer Inst. 2007;99:1232–9. https://doi.org/10.1093/jnci/djm086.

41. Dafer RM, Schneck M, Friberg TR, Jay WM. Intravitreal ranibizumab and bevacizumab: a review of risk. Semin Ophthalmol. 2007;22:201–4. https://doi.org/10.1080/08820530701543024.

42. Anderson KC. Lenalidomide and thalidomide: Mechanisms of action - Similarities and differences. Semin Hematol. 2005;S3–S8.

43. Wahl ML, Kenan DJ, Gonzalez-Gronow M, Pizzo SV. Angiostatin's molecular mechanism: aspects of specificity and regulation elucidated. J Cell Biochem. 2005;96:242–61. https://doi.org/10.1002/jcb.20480.

44. Thomas M, Kienast Y, Scheuer W, et al. A novel angiopoietin-2 selective fully human antibody with potent anti-tumoral and anti-angiogenic efficacy and superior side effect profile compared to Pan-Angiopoietin-1/-2 inhibitors. PLoS ONE. 2013;8:e54923. https://doi.org/10.1371/journal.pone.0054923.

45. Behl T, Kaur I, Goel H, Kotwani A. Significance of the antiangiogenic mechanisms of thalidomide in the therapy of diabetic retinopathy. Vascul Pharmacol. 2017;92:6–15. https://doi.org/10.1016/j.vph.2015.07.003.

46. Gössl M, Herrmann J, Tang H, et al. Prevention of vasa vasorum neovascularization attenuates early neointima formation in experimental hypercholesterolemia. Basic Res Cardiol. 2009;104:695–706. https://doi.org/10.1007/s00395-009-0036-0.

47. Kampschulte M, Gunkel I, Stieger P, et al. Thalidomide influences atherogenesis in aortas of ApoE$^{-/-}$/LDLR$^{-/-}$ double knockout mice: a nano-CT study. Int J Cardiovasc Imaging. 2014;30:795–802. https://doi.org/10.1007/s10554-014-0380-5.

48. Moser TL, Stack MS, Asplin I, et al. Angiostatin binds ATP synthase on the surface of human endothelial cells. Proc Natl Acad Sci USA. 1999;96:2811–6.

49. Moulton KS, Vakili K, Zurakowski D, et al. Inhibition of plaque neovascularization reduces macrophage accumulation and progression of advanced atherosclerosis. Proc Natl Acad Sci. 2003;100:4736–41. https://doi.org/10.1073/pnas.0730843100.

50. Moulton KS, Heller E, Konerding MA, et al. Angiogenesis inhibitors endostatin or TNP-470 reduce intimal neovascularization and plaque growth in apolipoprotein E-deficient mice. Circulation. 1999;99:1726–32.

51. Drinane M, Mollmark J, Zagorchev L, et al. The antiangiogenic activity of rPAI-1(23) inhibits vasa vasorum and growth of atherosclerotic plaque. Circ Res. 2009;104:337–45. https://doi.org/10.1161/CIRCRESAHA.108.184622.

52. Mollmark J, Ravi S, Sun B, et al. Antiangiogenic activity of rPAI-1(23) promotes vasa vasorum regression in hypercholesterolemic mice through a plasmin-dependent mechanism. Circ Res. 2011;108:1419–28. https://doi.org/10.1161/CIRCRESAHA.111.246249.

53. Mina R, Cerrato C, Bernardini A, et al. New pharmacotherapy options for multiple myeloma. Expert Opin Pharmacother. 2016;17:181–92. https://doi.org/10.1517/14656566.2016.1115016.

54. Rajabi M, Mousa S. The role of angiogenesis in cancer treatment. Biomedicines. 2017;5:34. https://doi.org/10.3390/biomedicines5020034.

55. Gullestad L, Ueland T, Fjeld JG, et al. Effect of thalidomide on cardiac remodeling in chronic heart failure: results of a double-blind, placebo-controlled study. Circulation. 2005;112:3408–14. https://doi.org/10.1161/CIRCULATIONAHA.105.564971.

56. Fernando NT, Koch M, Rothrock C, et al. Tumor escape from endogenous, extracellular matrix-associated angiogenesis inhibitors by up-regulation of multiple proangiogenic factors. Clin Cancer Res. 2008;14:1529–39. https://doi.org/10.1158/1078-0432. CCR-07-4126.

57. Pelaz B, Alexiou C, Alvarez-Puebla RA, et al. Diverse applications of nanomedicine. ACS Nano. 2017;11:2313–81. https://doi.org/10.1021/acsnano.6b06040.

58. Kipp JE. The role of solid nanoparticle technology in the parenteral delivery of poorly water-soluble drugs. Int J Pharm. 2004;284:109–22. https://doi.org/10.1016/j. ijpharm.2004.07.019.

59. Ofek P, Tiram G, Satchi-Fainaro R. Angiogenesis regulation by nanocarriers bearing RNA interference. Adv Drug Deliv Rev. 2017;119:3–19. https://doi.org/10.1016/j. addr.2017.01.008.

60. Niu Z, Conejos-Sánchez I, Griffin BT, et al. Lipid-based nanocarriers for oral peptide delivery. Adv Drug Deliv Rev. 2016;106:337–54. https://doi.org/10.1016/j. addr.2016.04.001.

61. Alaarg A, Pérez-Medina C, Metselaar JM, et al. Applying nanomedicine in maladaptive inflammation and angiogenesis. Adv Drug Deliv Rev. 2017;119:143–58. https://doi. org/10.1016/j.addr.2017.05.009.

62. Matoba T, Koga J, Nakano K, et al. Nanoparticle-mediated drug delivery system for atherosclerotic cardiovascular disease. J Cardiol. 2017;70:206–11. https://doi.org/10.1016/j. jjcc.2017.03.005.

63. Wang Y, Liu P, Duan Y, et al. Specific cell targeting with APRPG conjugated PEG-PLGA nanoparticles for treating ovarian cancer. Biomaterials. 2014;35:983–92. https://doi. org/10.1016/j.biomaterials.2013.09.062.

64. Winter PM, Caruthers SD, Zhang H, et al. Antiangiogenic synergism of integrin-targeted fumagillin nanoparticles and atorvastatin in atherosclerosis. JACC Cardiovasc Imaging. 2008;1:624–34. https://doi.org/10.1016/j.jcmg.2008.06.003.

65. Winter PM, Neubauer AM, Caruthers SD, et al. Endothelial alpha(v)beta3 integrin-targeted fumagillin nanoparticles inhibit angiogenesis in atherosclerosis. Arterioscler Thromb Vasc Biol. 2006;26:2103–9. https://doi.org/10.1161/01.ATV.0000235724.11299.76.

66. Katsuki S, Matoba T, Nakashiro S, et al. Nanoparticle-mediated delivery of pitavastatin inhibits atherosclerotic plaque destabilization/rupture in mice by regulating the recruitment of inflammatory monocytes. Circulation. 2014;129:896–906. https://doi.org/10.1161/ CIRCULATIONAHA.113.002870.

67. Nakashiro S, Matoba T, Umezu R, et al. Pioglitazone-incorporated nanoparticles prevent plaque destabilization and rupture by Regulating Monocyte/Macrophage Differentiation in ApoE$^{-/-}$ Mice. Arterioscler Thromb Vasc Biol. 2016;36:491–500. https://doi.org/10.1161/ ATVBAHA.115.307057.

68. Beldman TJ, Senders ML, Alaarg A, et al. Hyaluronan nanoparticles selectively target plaque-associated macrophages and improve plaque stability in atherosclerosis. ACS Nano. 2017;11:5785–99. https://doi.org/10.1021/acsnano.7b01385.

69. Sager HB, Dutta P, Dahlman JE, et al. RNAi targeting multiple cell adhesion molecules reduces immune cell recruitment and vascular inflammation after myocardial infarction. Sci Transl Med. 2016;8:342ra80–342ra80. https://doi.org/10.1126/scitranslmed.aaf1435.

70. Parvanian S, Mostafavi SM, Aghashiri M. Multifunctional nanoparticle developments in cancer diagnosis and treatment. Sens Bio-Sensing Res. 2017;13:81–7. https://doi. org/10.1016/J.SBSR.2016.08.002.

71. Tang J, Baxter S, Menon A, et al. Immune cell screening of a nanoparticle library improves atherosclerosis therapy. Proc Natl Acad Sci. 2016;113:E6731–40. https://doi. org/10.1073/pnas.1609629113.

72. De Bock K, Georgiadou M, Schoors S, et al. Role of PFKFB3-driven glycolysis in vessel sprouting. Cell. 2013;154:651–63. https://doi.org/10.1016/j.cell.2013.06.037.

73. Boyle EC, Sedding DG, Haverich A. Targeting vasa vasorum dysfunction to prevent atherosclerosis. Vascul Pharmacol. 2017;96–98:5–10. https://doi.org/10.1016/j.vph.2017.08.003.

74. Sedding DG, Boyle EC, Demandt JAF, et al. Vasa vasorum angiogenesis: key player in the initiation and progression of atherosclerosis and potential target for the treatment of cardiovascular disease. Front Immunol. 2018;9:706. https://doi.org/10.3389/fimmu.2018.00706.

75. Bierhansl L, Conradi L-C, Treps L, et al. Central role of metabolism in endothelial cell function and vascular disease. Physiology. 2017;32:126–40. https://doi.org/10.1152/physiol.00031.2016.

76. Missiaen R, Morales-Rodriguez F, Eelen G, Carmeliet P. Targeting endothelial metabolism for anti-angiogenesis therapy: a pharmacological perspective. Vascul Pharmacol. 2017;90:8–18. https://doi.org/10.1016/j.vph.2017.01.001.

77. Potente M, Carmeliet P. The link between angiogenesis and endothelial metabolism. Annu Rev Physiol. 2017;79:43–66. https://doi.org/10.1146/annurev-physiol-021115-105134.

78. Teuwen L-A, Draoui N, Dubois C, Carmeliet P. Endothelial cell metabolism. Curr Opin Hematol. 2017;24:240–7. https://doi.org/10.1097/MOH.0000000000000335.

79. Schoors S, De Bock K, Cantelmo AR, et al. Partial and transient reduction of glycolysis by PFKFB3 blockade reduces pathological angiogenesis. Cell Metab. 2014;19:37–48. https://doi.org/10.1016/j.cmet.2013.11.008.

80. Cantelmo AR, Conradi L-C, Brajic A, et al. Inhibition of the glycolytic activator PFKFB3 in endothelium induces tumor vessel normalization, impairs metastasis, and improves chemotherapy. Cancer Cell. 2016;30:968–85. https://doi.org/10.1016/j.ccell.2016.10.006.

81. Nakashima Y, Raines EW, Plump AS, et al. Upregulation of VCAM-1 and ICAM-1 at atherosclerosis-prone sites on the endothelium in the ApoE-deficient mouse. Arterioscler Thromb Vasc Biol. 1998;18:842–51.

82. O'Brien KD, Allen MD, McDonald TO, et al. Vascular cell adhesion molecule-1 is expressed in human coronary atherosclerotic plaques. Implications for the mode of progression of advanced coronary atherosclerosis. J Clin Invest. 1993;92:945–51. https://doi.org/10.1172/JCI116670.

83. O'Brien KD, McDonald TO, Chait A, et al. Neovascular expression of E-selectin, intercellular adhesion molecule-1, and vascular cell adhesion molecule-1 in human atherosclerosis and their relation to intimal leukocyte content. Circulation. 1996;93:672–82.

84. Ivanova EA, Bobryshev YV, Orekhov AN. Intimal pericytes as the second line of immune defence in atherosclerosis. World J Cardiol. 2015;7:583–93. https://doi.org/10.4330/wjc.v7.i10.583.

85. Ivanova E, Kovacs-Oller T, Sagdullaev BT. Vascular pericyte impairment and connexin43 gap junction deficit contribute to vasomotor decline in diabetic retinopathy. J Neurosci. 2017;37:7580–94. https://doi.org/10.1523/JNEUROSCI.0187-17.2017.

86. Schoors S, Cantelmo AR, Georgiadou M, et al. Incomplete and transitory decrease of glycolysis: a new paradigm for anti-angiogenic therapy? Cell Cycle. 2014;13:16–22. https://doi.org/10.4161/cc.27519.

87. Lapel M, Weston P, Strassheim D, et al. Glycolysis and oxidative phosphorylation are essential for purinergic receptor-mediated angiogenic responses in vasa vasorum endothelial cells. Am J Physiol Cell Physiol. 2017;312:C56–70. https://doi.org/10.1152/ajpcell.00250.2016.

88. Yegutkin GG, Helenius M, Kaczmarek E, et al. Chronic hypoxia impairs extracellular nucleotide metabolism and barrier function in pulmonary artery vasa vasorum endothelial cells. Angiogenesis. 2011;14:503–13. https://doi.org/10.1007/s10456-011-9234-0.

89. Brown JD, Lin CY, Duan Q, et al. NF-κB directs dynamic super enhancer formation in inflammation and atherogenesis. Mol Cell. 2014;56:219–31. https://doi.org/10.1016/j.molcel.2014.08.024.

90. Zaina S, Heyn H, Carmona FJ, et al. DNA methylation map of human atherosclerosis. Circ Cardiovasc Genet. 2014;7:692–700. https://doi.org/10.1161/CIRCGENETICS.113.000441.

91. Kumar A, Kumar S, Vikram A, et al. Histone and DNA methylation-mediated epigenetic downregulation of endothelial Kruppel-like factor 2 by low-density lipoprotein cholesterol. Arterioscler Thromb Vasc Biol. 2013;33:1936–42. https://doi.org/10.1161/ATVBAHA.113.301765.

92. Cao Q, Wang X, Jia L, et al. Inhibiting DNA Methylation by 5-Aza-2'-deoxycytidine ameliorates atherosclerosis through suppressing macrophage inflammation. Endocrinology. 2014;155:4925–38. https://doi.org/10.1210/en.2014-1595.

93. Dunn J, Qiu H, Kim S, et al. Flow-dependent epigenetic DNA methylation regulates endothelial gene expression and atherosclerosis. J Clin Invest. 2014;124:3187–99. https://doi.org/10.1172/JCI74792.

94. Ferri E, Petosa C, McKenna CE. Bromodomains: Structure, function and pharmacology of inhibition. Biochem Pharmacol. 2016;106:1–18. https://doi.org/10.1016/j.bcp.2015.12.005.

95. da Motta LL, Ledaki I, Purshouse K, et al. The BET inhibitor JQ1 selectively impairs tumour response to hypoxia and downregulates CA9 and angiogenesis in triple negative breast cancer. Oncogene. 2017;36:122–32. https://doi.org/10.1038/onc.2016.184.

96. Hosin AA, Prasad A, Viiri LE, et al. MicroRNAs in atherosclerosis. J Vasc Res. 2014;51:338–49. https://doi.org/10.1159/000368193.

97. Christopher A, Kaur R, Kaur G, et al. MicroRNA therapeutics: discovering novel targets and developing specific therapy. Perspect Clin Res. 2016;7:68. https://doi.org/10.4103/2229-3485.179431.

98. Araldi E, Chamorro-Jorganes A, van Solingen C, et al. Therapeutic potential of modulating microRNAs in atherosclerotic vascular disease. Curr Vasc Pharmacol. 2013.

99. Welten SMJ, Goossens EAC, Quax PHA, Nossent AY. The multifactorial nature of microRNAs in vascular remodelling. Cardiovasc Res. 2016;110:6–22. https://doi.org/10.1093/cvr/cvw039.

100. Harris TA, Yamakuchi M, Ferlito M, et al. MicroRNA-126 regulates endothelial expression of vascular cell adhesion molecule 1. Proc Natl Acad Sci USA. 2008;105:1516–21. https://doi.org/10.1073/pnas.0707493105.

101. Fish JE, Santoro MM, Morton SU, et al. miR-126 regulates angiogenic signaling and vascular integrity. Dev Cell. 2008;15:272–84. https://doi.org/10.1016/j.devcel.2008.07.008.

102. van Solingen C, Seghers L, Bijkerk R, et al. Antagomir-mediated silencing of endothelial cell specific microRNA-126 impairs ischemia-induced angiogenesis. J Cell Mol Med. 2009;13:1577–85. https://doi.org/10.1111/j.1582-4934.2008.00613.x.

103. Voellenkle C, van Rooij J, Guffanti A, et al. Deep-sequencing of endothelial cells exposed to hypoxia reveals the complexity of known and novel microRNAs. RNA. 2012;18:472–84. https://doi.org/10.1261/rna.027615.111.

104. Chistiakov DA, Sobenin IA, Orekhov AN, Bobryshev YV. Human miR-221/222 in physiological and atherosclerotic vascular remodeling. Biomed Res Int. 2015;2015:1–18. https://doi.org/10.1155/2015/354517.

105. Suarez Y, Fernandez-Hernando C, Pober JS, Sessa WC. Dicer dependent microRNAs regulate gene expression and functions in human endothelial cells. Circ Res. 2007;100:1164–73. https://doi.org/10.1161/01.RES.0000265065.26744.17.

106. Liu X, Cheng Y, Zhang S, et al. A necessary role of miR-221 and miR-222 in vascular smooth muscle cell proliferation and neointimal hyperplasia. Circ Res. 2009;104:476–87. https://doi.org/10.1161/CIRCRESAHA.108.185363.

107. Janssen HLA, Reesink HW, Lawitz EJ, et al. Treatment of HCV infection by targeting microRNA. N Engl J Med. 2013;368:1685–94. https://doi.org/10.1056/NEJMoa1209026.

108. Jäckel S, Kiouptsi K, Lillich M, et al. Gut microbiota regulate hepatic von Willebrand factor synthesis and arterial thrombus formation via Toll-like receptor-2. Blood. 2017;130:542–53. https://doi.org/10.1182/blood-2016-11-754416.

109. Spadoni I, Zagato E, Bertocchi A, et al. A gut-vascular barrier controls the systemic dissemination of bacteria. Science. 2015;350:830–4. https://doi.org/10.1126/science.aad0135.

110. Wang Z, Roberts AB, Buffa JA, et al. Non-lethal inhibition of gut microbial trimethylamine production for the treatment of atherosclerosis. Cell. 2015;163:1585–95. https://doi.org/10.1016/j.cell.2015.11.055.

111. Roberts AB, Gu X, Buffa JA, et al. Development of a gut microbe-targeted nonlethal therapeutic to inhibit thrombosis potential. Nat Med. 2018;24:1407–17. https://doi.org/10.1038/s41591-018-0128-1.

Chapter 7
Supporting Microvasculature Function

7.1 Why Describing Atherosclerosis as a Microvasculature Disease is Important

What are we missing when we overlook the role of the microvascular in atherosclerosis? When the microvasculature is not considered, fundamental aspects of disease progression are ignored and potential key targets for prevention and therapeutic intervention are left unexploited. The dogma in the atherosclerosis field states that it is the endothelium lining of the medium and large conduit arteries that is first compromised during disease development. For this reason, and due to the ease of isolation, the majority of atherosclerosis research on endothelial cells has focused on macrovascular endothelial cells. Yet as we've contended in this book, atherosclerosis actually begins in the vessel wall microvasculature. Importantly, **there are substantial structural, functional, and site-specific differences between micro- and macrovascular endothelial cells** [1–3]. For example, they differ in their barrier function [4–6], gene expression patterns [7, 8], signal transduction networks [9], and consequently, their responsiveness and vulnerability to inflammatory stimuli [1, 10, 11]. Acknowledging the heterogeneity of endothelial cell populations should spur research into the phenotype and signaling pathways occurring specifically in diseased and healthy microvascular endothelial cells which could then be exploited for targeted drug intervention. In this case, anatomically restricted expression of molecular signatures would facilitate selective drug targeting to diseased microvascular endothelial cell populations. For example, drug cargo could be homed to vasa vasorum using antibodies or peptides specific for adhesion molecules, integrins, or growth factor receptors upregulated in dysfunctional vasa vasorum endothelial cells. Moreover, acknowledgment of the role of the microvasculature opens atherosclerosis researchers to the expansive field of pathological angiogenesis and to the potential repurposing of the drugs and therapeutic strategies designed for cancer and inflammation treatment.

© Springer Nature Switzerland AG 2019
A. Haverich and E. C. Boyle, *Atherosclerosis Pathogenesis and Microvascular Dysfunction*, https://doi.org/10.1007/978-3-030-20245-3_7

Therefore, changing the mind-set of clinicians and researchers in the field of atherosclerosis to reconsider the importance of the arterial wall microvasculature is crucial if we are to come closer to preventing and treating this deadly disease.

7.2 Missing Pieces in the Site-Specificity Puzzle

In Chap. 4, we emphasized that atherosclerosis demonstrates significant site specificity, with hot spots of disease development while other sites are nearly always disease-free. We made the case for an outside-in development of disease emphasizing the role of vasa vasorum and lymphatic microvessel dysfunction. In particular, microvascular dysfunction correlates with many different stages of disease development from initiation to destabilization of the plaque. Yet, even within a diseased artery itself, plaques are often eccentric leading to an important question: what makes one side of an artery more susceptible to disease—or conversely— what protects the other side from disease in the face of systemic inflammatory insults or all other risk factors? One idea could be that the asymmetrical distribution of lymphatic vessels or lymph nodes contributes to site-specific adventitial inflammation. Clues from the locoregional deposition of bacteria in atherosclerotic plaques (e.g., own mouth bacteria in carotid artery plaques [12–14], own leg/feet bacteria in femoral artery plaques [15–17]) suggests there may be an early role of impaired lymphatic clearance of bacteria in disease initiation. Looking at the type of microbes involved in mycotic aneurysms, we would like to note an interesting locoregional preference of aneurysms in the chest, abdomen, peripheral arteries, and cerebral circulation. Bacteria from the oral cavity have been found in up to 70% of all intracerebral aneurysms [18]. Inflammatory aneurysms of the abdominal aorta, by contrast, exhibit contamination by enteric bacteria in a significant proportion of subjects [19, 20]. In thoracic aortic aneurysms, a mixed picture exists. In the specific case of syphilitic aneurysm, *Treponema pallidum* only very rarely affects sites other than thoracic segments of the aorta. Here, pathologists have clearly identified the outside-in route of infection from the lung, via the pulmonary lymphatics, to the aortic adventitia. From there, *T. pallidum* shows a particular predilection toward vasa vasorum of the aortic wall, leading to their occlusion via inflammatory processes [21–23]. Yet, compared to blood vessels, studying the lymphatic microvasculature is inherently difficult although increasing genetic tools and transgenic mice are making progress in this area.

Another potential aggravator of vasa vasorum dysfunction is the perivascular adipose tissue (PVAT) that surrounds and penetrates the adventitia. Under physiological conditions, PVAT regulates vascular homeostasis and has potent antiatherogenic properties. In contrast, under certain pathological conditions (e.g., diabetes, obesity), PVAT becomes dysfunctional secreting pro-inflammatory adipokines that induce endothelial dysfunction and stimulate the recruitment of inflammatory cells [24]. The distribution and phenotype of PVAT have been suggested to also play a role in the development of atherosclerosis [25], but we would specifically argue that, as opposed to its effects on the luminal endothelium, its more consequential effects are on the adventitial microvasculature.

7.3 Supporting Microvasculature Function to Enable Atherosclerosis Regression

Regression of established atherosclerotic disease is an obvious and long sought-after therapeutic goal. Regression can include a decrease in plaque volume and/or a change in plaque composition to a less inflammatory, less lipid-laden form. There is substantial evidence from animal studies that even advanced atherosclerotic plaques can regress [26]. Facilitating this work is the fact that regression in animals can be examined post mortem by analyzing vessel wall lipid content, thickness, and cellular composition. **Whether in mouse, rabbit, pig, or nonhuman primate models of atherosclerosis, successful regression almost always requires drastic improvements in previously non-physiologically high plasma lipid profiles.** This can be achieved by changing the animals' diets, or in the case of atherosclerosis mouse models, adenoviral-mediated gene transfer of *apoE* in ApoE$^{-/-}$ mice or *ldlr* in Ldlr$^{-/-}$ mice. Regression is characterized by intensive plaque remodeling including a reduction in lipid content and necrotic core area and an enrichment of alternatively activated, anti-inflammatory, tissue-remodeling M2 macrophages [26, 27].

Whether human atherosclerotic plaques are capable of regressing has been controversial over the years [28–30]. One major criticism has been whether it's possible to sufficiently distinguish between a slowing of disease progression and bona fide disease regression. In humans, the evaluation of regression has relied primarily on angiography or intravascular ultrasonography which measure luminal stenosis and wall thickness, respectively. Results from large lipid-lowering clinical trials revealed very small but significant reductions (<1%) in stenosis alongside very large reductions in coronary events [31]. This is proposed to be because the plaques most vulnerable to thrombosis actually exhibit less than 50% stenosis and that remodeling during regression very likely involves stabilization of the smaller, more vulnerable plaques [32]. Future progress into imaging modalities that assess compositional changes to the blood vessel wall (e.g., near infrared spectroscopy) will allow better assessment of regression of atherosclerosis upon therapeutic intervention.

Both the blood and lymphatic microvasculature likely play a vital role in regression of atherosclerotic plaques. In the case of leaky vasa vasorum, one of the first steps in regression must be to halt the further deposition of atherogenic substances into the vessel wall by restoring the integrity of leaky vasa vasorum. Aggressive lowering of plasma lipids is simply not sufficient if inflammatory processes weaken the microcirculatory endothelial barrier. By analogy, just because it has stopped raining, doesn't mean the roof is not still leaky! As has been shown time and time again, a majority of high-risk atherosclerosis patients on aggressive statin therapy have a residual inflammatory risk for cardiovascular events [33].

Therefore, to reestablish the integrity of the vascular wall microcirculatory beds, inflammation must also be aggressively reduced.

Another key step in regression is the removal of cholesterol and emigration of monocyte-derived cells (including lipid-laden foam cells) from plaques. This requires proper-functioning vessel wall lymphatic vessels which are present not only in the adventitia but also reach into the intima [34, 35]. Lymphatic vessels were shown in an animal model to play an important role in reverse cholesterol transport (RCT) from atherosclerotic plaques [36]. When plaque-laden aortic arches with stable isotope-labeled cholesterol were transplanted into recipient mice, efflux of cholesterol out of the plaque was evident only when mice were treated with a control antibody. Conversely, if lymphatic regrowth was blocked with an anti-VEGFR3 antibody, cholesterol was retained in the plaque [37]. To facilitate better clearance of lipids by the lymphatic microvasculature, new efforts are being put into increasing the solubility of cholesterol crystals. Cyclic oligosaccharide 2-hydroxypropyl-β-cyclodextrin (CD) is a compound that increases solubility of cholesterol and is approved for human use for the delivery of lipophilic drugs. In mice, CD can prevent and reverse established atherosclerosis, even in the face of a continued cholesterol-rich diet [38]. Repurposing of CD to dissolve extra- and intracellular cholesterol crystals and increase RCT out of the atheroma could be effective in aiding regression.

Cellular senescence is a stress response characterized by irreversible cell cycle arrest resulting in loss of tissue-repair capabilities. Senescent cells display a so-called senescence-associated secretory phenotype characterized by the secretion of pro-inflammatory and matrix-degrading molecules. Advanced atherosclerotic lesions contain senescent endothelial cells and vascular smooth muscle cells which are thought to induce chronic sterile inflammation and vascular remodeling that contributes to plaque development and instability [39–41]. In animal models of atherosclerosis, selective clearance of senescent cells is atheroprotective [42, 43]. Accordingly, there is increasing interest in senolytic therapies to remove senescence cells to not only prevent but also regress, atherosclerosis. Aged hypercholesterolemic mice with preexisting plaques showed improved endothelial function and significantly reduced plaque calcification with chronic senolytic treatment [43]. And while overall plaque burden and composition were not affected, these **senolytic drugs may prove to be complementary to lipid-lowering and anti-inflammatory concepts especially when tackling particularly recalcitrant plaques.**

7.4   Beyond Risk Factors: Lifestyle Factors to Maintain a Competent Vessel Wall Microvasculature

In Chap. 2, we reviewed the classical risk factors for atherosclerosis development. Yet it's interesting that there a large percentage of individuals with clinically significant atherosclerosis that do not appear to have any classical risk factors [44, 45].

What advice can we offer these individuals? What are some everyday things one can do to keep your microvasculature healthy? **Ideally, one would want to prevent vasa vasorum occlusion and leakiness, promote endothelial repair processes through stimulation of bone marrow-derived and vascular resident endothelial stem cells, and support lymphatic clearance of lipids and inflammatory cells out of the plaque.** Exercise, as we covered in Sect. 5.4, is a very effective way to ensure microvascular health, to not only prevent and treat atherosclerosis but also other microvascular-related diseases. Now we'd like to discuss the evidence for the effect of two more lifestyle factors on atherosclerosis and suggest they could be incorporated into both primary and secondary prevention of cardiovascular disease.

7.4.1   Sleep

Too little sleep is associated with an increased risk of all-cause mortality and cardiovascular events [46, 47]. Short sleep duration is also associated with carotid intima–media thickness, a noninvasive measure of atherosclerosis [48]. **Mechanistically, the link between sleep and cardiovascular disease is thought to be in large part due to the detrimental effects of short sleep duration on vascular function.** Habitual short sleep time (≤ 6 hours) as well as acute (≥ 24 hours) or partial (≤ 5 hours) sleep deprivation has been shown to raise blood pressure, increase systemic inflammation, and impair endothelial function [49, 50]. Nightshift workers in particular are known to have reduced endothelial function [51] and be at higher risk of cardiovascular disease [52, 53]. In interventional studies on healthy subjects, sleep loss significantly increases circulating levels of endothelial activation markers (e.g., E-selectin and ICAM-1) and pro-inflammatory cytokines (e.g., TNFα, IL-1β, IL-6) [54, 55].

Indeed, dramatic changes in gene expression occur following short sleep duration [56, 57]. As gene expression can be regulated by epigenetic mechanisms, epigenetic alterations that occur following insufficient sleep are of interest as they may be a mechanistic link between sleep loss and atherosclerosis development. In both animal studies and humans, sleep loss has been shown to impact the three primary epigenetic mechanisms: (i) DNA methylation, (ii) histone modifications, and (iii) noncoding RNAs [58]. This field of research is relatively new and a better understanding of the effects of sleep on the epigenetic landscape is needed. In particular, more research is needed to identify and link the genes affected by sleep loss-induced epigenetic modifications to pathomechanisms of atherosclerosis development, with particular emphasis on inflammation and the microvasculature.

Sleep loss has also been causally linked with the molecular processes involved in cellular senescence. One extraordinary example of the effect of chronic short sleep duration on cellular senescence came from data collected in the large prospective Nurses' Health Study cohort. This study examined senescence by measuring telomere length. In women under 50 years old who slept ≤ 6 hours/day, compared to ≥ 9 hours/day, the equivalent of a 9-year telomere attrition in their peripheral blood leukocytes was observed. In another study of older adults, partial sleep deprivation (1 night of 4 hours of sleep) activated the DNA damage response and senescence-associated secretory phenotype in peripheral blood leukocytes. The importance of cellular senescence during atherosclerosis development is becoming more apparent. Therefore, understanding the biological mechanisms that link short sleep duration to cellular aging will provide us with a better grasp of how sleep duration and atherosclerosis are related.

Several studies have looked specifically at the effects of sleep duration on the microvasculature. For example, in healthy middle-aged individuals, self-reported sleep quality and duration were inversely related to microvascular function [59]. Sauvet et al. (2010) found that acute sleep deprivation of 40 hours caused a significant decrease in microvascular reactivity reflecting hypoperfusion of the microvasculature [60]. In healthy male volunteers, coronary microcirculation was impaired after a single night of 4 hours sleep compared to 7 hours [61]. Similarly, female nurses after a single night shift also displayed impaired coronary microcirculation [62]. To date, there have been no studies on the effect of sleep loss on vasa vasorum in particular, but one could easily imagine their structure and function being similarly affected by the aforementioned mediators (e.g., inflammation, high blood pressure). Therefore, it's hypothesized that, in the acute case, sleep deprivation might serve as a trigger for cardiovascular events. In the case of repetitive short sleep duration, the resultant chronic vascular dysfunction, inflammation, and high blood pressure likely affect the vasa vasorum, and thereby could contribute to atherosclerosis development.

The brain has a unique mechanism to achieve fluid balance, interstitial waste removal, and lipid transport. This so-called glymphatic pathway is a glial cell-dependent perivascular network that serves a pseudo-lymphatic function [63]. Cerebrospinal fluid enters the brain via this pathway and flows along arterial perivascular spaces into the brain interstitium, driving perivenous drainage of interstitial fluid and its solutes [64]. The flow of cerebrospinal fluid into the glymphatic pathway is driven by arterial pulsations [65], but intriguingly, primarily functions during sleep [66]. Impaired glymphatic flow leads to reduced clearance of waste products (e.g., amyloid-beta) and intracellular lipid accumulation. Sleep deprivation in mice causes sharp reductions in glymphatic clearance of interstitial solutes [67, 68]. As sleep is an important regulator of glymphatic flow and lack of sleep is a risk factor for cardiovascular disease, it would interesting in the future to study whether short sleep duration could contribute to atherosclerosis development in the brain (leading to stroke) by increasing perivascular inflammation.

7.4.2 Vaccination

It was first observed in the early 1930s that influenza epidemics track closely with spikes in cardiovascular mortality [68]. Today, it is well established that recent influenza infection is associated with both fatal and nonfatal atherothrombotic events [69, 70]. A recent study calculated the risk of myocardial infarction during the week after laboratory-confirmed infection with influenza virus to be 6 times higher than the year before or after diagnosis [71]. **Evidence from cohort studies and randomized clinical trials indicate that the influenza vaccine is effective in preventing cardiovascular events and all-cause mortality, especially in patients with preexisting cardiovascular disease** [72–74]. A meta-analysis of five randomized trials showed a 36% lower risk of major adverse cardiovascular events among adults who had received an influenza vaccine that season compared to those who had not [75].

Epidemiological data also strongly suggests that *Streptococcus pneumoniae* infection is a potential risk factor for adverse cardiovascular events, especially in high-risk patients. It's estimated that patients have a fourfold higher risk of myocardial infarction, stroke, and fatal coronary heart disease in the first 30 days after hospitalization for pneumonia and this risk remains elevated during long-term follow-up [76, 77]. The evidence for a protective effect of pneumococcal vaccination on cardiovascular events relies primarily on retrospective observational studies [78]. To date, there have been no prospective randomized clinical trials evaluating the effect of pneumococcal vaccination on the clinical course of cardiovascular disease—studies that are urgently needed.

Varicella zoster virus (VZV) causes the common childhood infection known as chickenpox. Reactivation of the dormant virus later in life causes herpes zoster (also known as shingles). There is an accumulating body of evidence that herpes zoster is associated with an increased risk of cardio/cerebrovascular events [79–81]. Herpes zoster vaccines are relatively new and the low number of vaccinated individuals has limited the study of the role of this vaccine in prevention of cardiovascular and/or cerebrovascular events. Hopefully, with more health agencies and primary caregivers recommending older adults to be vaccinated against VZV [82], a clearer picture of its potential to reduce cardio/cerebrovascular events will emerge. **Therefore, influenza, pneumococcal, and VZC vaccination should be highly recommended for both primary prevention of cardiovascular disease and as part of comprehensive secondary prevention for at-risk individuals.**

7.4.3   Reducing Exposure to Air Pollution

As covered in Sect. 2.4.1, the association between air pollution and atherosclerosis is clear. Therefore, minimizing exposure to air pollution is a key way to reduce the burden of cardiovascular disease. When considering global particulate matter exposure, the magnitude of exposure to household sources of air pollution far outweighs ambient (outdoor) exposure. Approximately, 76% of all global particulate matter air pollution exposure occurs indoors in the developing world [83], coming primarily from burning biomass such as wood, charcoal, or dung for cooking, lighting, and heating. In this case, interventions to reduce indoor exposure include improving ventilation, separating cooking from other living areas, and replacing traditional methods of cooking with cleaner alternatives [84]. When we think about household personal exposure in the developed world, indoor-generated pollutant sources include cooking/frying, wood burning, tobacco smoke, cleaning detergents, as well as the burning of incense and candles. In the developed world, it's estimated that people spend 90% of their lives indoors with 70% of their daily time spent at home [85]. Accordingly, relatively simple changes to one's awareness and at home behaviors can significantly reduce personal exposure to harmful pollutants, and consequently, lower the risk of cardiovascular disease.

Individuals can also reduce their exposure to outdoor sources of air pollution. If possible, on days when the reported air pollution conditions are especially bad, one can avoid, or at least minimize, going outside or opening windows. Exercise outdoors when air pollution levels are high is also not recommended as it can increase the effective inhaled dose. For example, in a study of healthy adults, the dose of deposited particulate air pollution increased fivefold when performing moderate exercise compared to being at rest [86]. Of course, there is a risk/benefit analysis to be made from the positive health benefits of outdoor activity with the detrimental effects of breathing in air pollution. Encouraging individuals to exercise when and where (e.g., away from major roads) air pollution levels are lower may help to preserve the net positive benefits of exercise. Lastly, cleaning indoor air is another way in which personal exposure can be reduced. In two randomized, blinded, crossover studies looking at the effect of home high-efficiency particulate air filters on the microvasculature of healthy individuals, a significant improvement in microvascular function was observed [87, 88]. Thus, **filtering indoor air could also be used in primary and secondary prevention for atherosclerosis,** especially in at-risk populations (e.g., individuals living in highly polluted locations or having other underlying risk factors).

7.5 Concluding Remarks

Prevention is often a neglected field in medicine with the focus more often being on treatment of the disease after the fact. As outlined in this chapter, a few key behavioral lifestyle factors like getting enough sleep, getting vaccinated, avoiding air pollution exposure, and of course, exercise can really help prevent atherosclerosis. We argue that maintaining competent microvasculature, both blood and lymphatic, is fundamental in all aspects of atherosclerosis prevention.

References

1. Molema G. Heterogeneity in endothelial responsiveness to cytokines, molecular causes, and pharmacological consequences. Semin Thromb Hemost. 2010;36:246–64. https://doi.org/10.1055/s-0030-1253448.
2. Nolan DJ, Ginsberg M, Israely E, et al. Molecular signatures of tissue-specific microvascular endothelial cell heterogeneity in organ maintenance and regeneration. Dev Cell. 2013;26:204–19. https://doi.org/10.1016/j.devcel.2013.06.017.
3. Stevens T. Functional and molecular heterogeneity of pulmonary endothelial cells. Proc Am Thorac Soc. 2011;8:453–7. https://doi.org/10.1513/pats.201101-004MW.
4. Ofori-Acquah SF, King J, Voelkel N, et al. Heterogeneity of barrier function in the lung reflects diversity in endothelial cell junctions. Microvasc Res. 2008;75:391–402. https://doi.org/10.1016/j.mvr.2007.10.006.
5. Kelly JJ, Moore TM, Babal P, et al. Pulmonary microvascular and macrovascular endothelial cells: differential regulation of Ca^{2+} and permeability. Am J Physiol. 1998;274:L810–9.
6. Gündüz D, Aslam M, Krieger U, et al. Opposing effects of ATP and adenosine on barrier function of rat coronary microvasculature. J Mol Cell Cardiol. 2012;52:962–70. https://doi.org/10.1016/j.yjmcc.2012.01.003.
7. Jackson CJ, Nguyen M. Human microvascular endothelial cells differ from macrovascular endothelial cells in their expression of matrix metalloproteinases. Int J Biochem Cell Biol. 1997;29:1167–77.
8. Chi J-T, Chang HY, Haraldsen G, et al. Endothelial cell diversity revealed by global expression profiling. Proc Natl Acad Sci USA. 2003;100:10623–8. https://doi.org/10.1073/pnas.1434429100.
9. Moore TM, Chetham PM, Kelly JJ, Stevens T. Signal transduction and regulation of lung endothelial cell permeability. Interaction between calcium and cAMP. Am J Physiol. 1998;275:L203–22.
10. Viemann D, Goebeler M, Schmid S, et al. TNF induces distinct gene expression programs in microvascular and macrovascular human endothelial cells. J Leukoc Biol. 2006;80:174–85. https://doi.org/10.1189/jlb.0905530.
11. Gräfe M, Auch-Schwelk W, Hertel H, et al. Human cardiac microvascular and macrovascular endothelial cells respond differently to oxidatively modified LDL. Atherosclerosis. 1998;137:87–95.
12. Chhibber-Goel J, Singhal V, Bhowmik D, et al. Linkages between oral commensal bacteria and atherosclerotic plaques in coronary artery disease patients. NPJ Biofilms Microbiomes. 2016;2:7. https://doi.org/10.1038/s41522-016-0009-7.
13. Eberhard J, Stumpp N, Winkel A, et al. Streptococcus mitis and Gemella haemolysans were simultaneously found in atherosclerotic and oral plaques of elderly without periodontitis-a pilot study. Clin Oral Investig. 2017;21:447–52. https://doi.org/10.1007/s00784-016-1811-6.
14. Fernandes CP, Oliveira FA, Silva PG, et al. Molecular analysis of oral bacteria in dental biofilm and atherosclerotic plaques of patients with vascular disease. Int J Cardiol. 2014;174:710–2. https://doi.org/10.1016/j.ijcard.2014.04.201.
15. Snow DE, Everett J, Mayer G, et al. The presence of biofilm structures in atherosclerotic plaques of arteries from legs amputated as a complication of diabetic foot ulcers. J Wound Care 2016;25:S16–22. https://doi.org/10.12968/jowc.2016.25.Sup2.S16.
16. Olszewski WL, Rutkowska J, Moscicka-Wesolowska M, et al. Bacteria of leg atheromatous arteries responsible for inflammation. Vasa. 2016;45:379–85. https://doi.org/10.1024/0301-1526/a000549.
17. Andziak P, Olszewski WL, Moscicka-Wesolowska M, et al. Skin own bacteria may aggravate inflammatory and occlusive changes in atherosclerotic arteries of lower limbs. Int Angiol. 2012;31:474–82.
18. Peshkova IO, Schaefer G, Koltsova EK. Atherosclerosis and aortic aneurysm-is inflammation a common denominator? FEBS J. 2016;283:1636–52. https://doi.org/10.1111/febs.13634.

19. Johnsen SH, Forsdahl SH, Singh K, Jacobsen BK. Atherosclerosis in abdominal aortic aneurysms: a causal event or a process running in parallel? The Tromsø study. Arterioscler Thromb Vasc Biol. 2010;30:1263–8. https://doi.org/10.1161/ATVBAHA.110.203588.
20. Sterpetti AV, Feldhaus RJ, Schultz RD, Blair EA. Identification of abdominal aortic aneurysm patients with different clinical features and clinical outcomes. Am J Surg. 1988;156:466–9.
21. Martin H. Recherches sur la nature et la pathogénie des lésions viscérales consécutives à l'endartérite oblitérante et progressive. Scléroses dystrophiques. Rev méd. 1881;1:369.
22. Nakata Y, Shionoya S. Vascular lesions due to obstruction of the vasa vasorum. Nature. 1966;212:1258–9.
23. Reuter K. Neue befunde von Spirochaeta Pallida in menschlichen Körper und ihre Bedeutung für die Aetiologie der Syphilis. Zeitschrift für Hyg und Infekt. 1906;54:49–60.
24. Qi X-Y, Qu S-L, Xiong W-H, et al. Perivascular adipose tissue (PVAT) in atherosclerosis: a double-edged sword. Cardiovasc Diabetol. 2018;17:134. https://doi.org/10.1186/s12933-018-0777-x.
25. Tanaka K, Sata M. Roles of perivascular adipose tissue in the pathogenesis of atherosclerosis. Front Physiol. 2018;9:3. https://doi.org/10.3389/fphys.2018.00003.
26. Rahman K, Fisher EA. Insights from pre-clinical and clinical studies on the role of innate inflammation in atherosclerosis regression. Front Cardiovasc Med. 2018;5:32. https://doi.org/10.3389/fcvm.2018.00032.
27. Rahman K, Vengrenyuk Y, Ramsey SA, et al. Inflammatory Ly6Chi monocytes and their conversion to M2 macrophages drive atherosclerosis regression. J Clin Invest. 2017;127:2904–15. https://doi.org/10.1172/JCI75005.
28. Stein Y, Stein O. Does therapeutic intervention achieve slowing of progression or bona fide regression of atherosclerotic lesions? Arterioscler Thromb Vasc Biol. 2001;21:183–8.
29. Kunz J. Can atherosclerosis regress? The role of the vascular extracellular matrix and the age-related changes of arteries. Gerontology. 48:267–78. https://doi.org/10.1159/000065248.
30. Keraliya A, Blankstein R. Regression of coronary atherosclerosis with medical therapy. N Engl J Med. 2017;376:1370. https://doi.org/10.1056/NEJMicm1609054.
31. Brown BG, Zhao XQ, Sacco DE, Albers JJ. Lipid lowering and plaque regression. New insights into prevention of plaque disruption and clinical events in coronary disease. Circulation. 1993;87:1781–91.
32. Farmer JA, Gotto AM. Dyslipidemia and the vulnerable plaque. Prog Cardiovasc Dis. 44:415–28.
33. Ridker PM. How common is residual inflammatory risk? Circ Res. 2017;120:617–9. https://doi.org/10.1161/CIRCRESAHA.116.310527.
34. Nakano T, Nakashima Y, Yonemitsu Y, et al. Angiogenesis and lymphangiogenesis and expression of lymphangiogenic factors in the atherosclerotic intima of human coronary arteries. Hum Pathol. 2005;36:330–40. https://doi.org/10.1016/j.humpath.2005.01.001.
35. Zhang Y, Cliff WJ, Schoefl GI, Higgins G. Immunohistochemical study of intimal microvessels in coronary atherosclerosis. Am J Pathol. 1993;143:164–72.
36. Martel C, Li W, Fulp B, et al. Lymphatic vasculature mediates macrophage reverse cholesterol transport in mice. J Clin Invest. 2013;123:1571–9. https://doi.org/10.1172/JCI63685.
37. Llodra J, Angeli V, Liu J, et al. Emigration of monocyte-derived cells from atherosclerotic lesions characterizes regressive, but not progressive, plaques. Proc Natl Acad Sci USA. 2004;101:11779–84. https://doi.org/10.1073/pnas.0403259101.
38. Zimmer S, Grebe A, Bakke SS, et al. Cyclodextrin promotes atherosclerosis regression via macrophage reprogramming. Sci Transl Med. 2016;8:333ra50. https://doi.org/10.1126/scitranslmed.aad6100.
39. Minamino T, Miyauchi H, Yoshida T, et al. Endothelial cell senescence in human atherosclerosis: role of telomere in endothelial dysfunction. Circulation. 2002;105:1541–4.
40. Wang J, Uryga AK, Reinhold J, et al. Vascular smooth muscle cell senescence promotes atherosclerosis and features of plaque vulnerability. Circulation. 2015;132:1909–19. https://doi.org/10.1161/CIRCULATIONAHA.115.016457.

41. Gardner SE, Humphry M, Bennett MR, Clarke MCH. Senescent vascular smooth muscle cells drive inflammation through an Interleukin-1α-dependent senescence-associated secretory phenotype. Arterioscler Thromb Vasc Biol. 2015;35:1963–74. https://doi.org/10.1161/ATVBAHA.115.305896.

42. Childs BG, Baker DJ, Wijshake T, et al. Senescent intimal foam cells are deleterious at all stages of atherosclerosis. Science. 2016;354:472–7. https://doi.org/10.1126/science.aaf6659.

43. Roos CM, Zhang B, Palmer AK, et al. Chronic senolytic treatment alleviates established vasomotor dysfunction in aged or atherosclerotic mice. Aging Cell. 2016;15:973–7. https://doi.org/10.1111/acel.12458.

44. Baber U, Halperin JL. Variability in low-density lipoprotein cholesterol and cardiovascular risk: should consistency be a new target? J Am Coll Cardiol. 2015;65:1549–51.

45. Wilkins JT, Ning H, Berry J, et al. Lifetime risk and years lived free of total cardiovascular disease. JAMA. 2012;308:1795. https://doi.org/10.1001/jama.2012.14312.

46. Yin J, Jin X, Shan Z, et al. Relationship of sleep duration with all-cause mortality and cardiovascular events: a systematic review and dose-response meta-analysis of prospective cohort studies. J Am Heart Assoc. 2017;6. https://doi.org/10.1161/JAHA.117.005947.

47. Cappuccio FP, Cooper D, D'Elia L, et al. Sleep duration predicts cardiovascular outcomes: a systematic review and meta-analysis of prospective studies. Eur Heart J. 2011;32:1484–92. https://doi.org/10.1093/eurheartj/ehr007.

48. Wolff B, Völzke H, Schwahn C, et al. Relation of self-reported sleep duration with carotid intima-media thickness in a general population sample. Atherosclerosis. 2008;196:727–32. https://doi.org/10.1016/j.atherosclerosis.2006.12.023.

49. Pepin J-L, Borel A-L, Tamisier R, et al. Hypertension and sleep: overview of a tight relationship. Sleep Med Rev. 2014;18:509–19. https://doi.org/10.1016/j.smrv.2014.03.003.

50. Tobaldini E, Fiorelli EM, Solbiati M, et al. Short sleep duration and cardiometabolic risk: from pathophysiology to clinical evidence. Nat Rev Cardiol. 2018. https://doi.org/10.1038/s41569-018-0109-6.

51. Suessenbacher A, Potocnik M, Dörler J, et al. Comparison of peripheral endothelial function in shift versus nonshift workers. Am J Cardiol. 2011;107:945–8. https://doi.org/10.1016/j.amjcard.2010.10.077.

52. Vetter C, Devore EE, Wegrzyn LR, et al. Association between rotating night shift work and risk of coronary heart disease among women. JAMA. 2016;315:1726–34. https://doi.org/10.1001/jama.2016.4454.

53. Kawachi I, Colditz GA, Stampfer MJ, et al. Prospective study of shift work and risk of coronary heart disease in women. Circulation. 1995;92:3178–82.

54. Mullington JM, Simpson NS, Meier-Ewert HK, Haack M. Sleep loss and inflammation. Best Pract Res Clin Endocrinol Metab. 2010;24:775–84. https://doi.org/10.1016/j.beem.2010.08.014.

55. Mullington JM, Haack M, Toth M, et al. Cardiovascular, inflammatory, and metabolic consequences of sleep deprivation. Prog Cardiovasc Dis. 2009;51:294–302. https://doi.org/10.1016/j.pcad.2008.10.003.

56. Cirelli C, Tononi G. Differences in gene expression during sleep and wakefulness. Ann Med. 1999;31:117–24.

57. Archer SN, Oster H. How sleep and wakefulness influence circadian rhythmicity: effects of insufficient and mistimed sleep on the animal and human transcriptome. J Sleep Res. 2015;24:476–93. https://doi.org/10.1111/jsr.12307.

58. Gaine ME, Chatterjee S, Abel T. Sleep deprivation and the epigenome. Front Neural Circuits. 2018;12:14. https://doi.org/10.3389/fncir.2018.00014.

59. Bonsen T, Wijnstok NJ, Hoekstra T, et al. Sleep quality and duration are related to microvascular function: the Amsterdam Growth and Health Longitudinal Study. J Sleep Res. 2015;24:140–7. https://doi.org/10.1111/jsr.12256.

60. Sauvet F, Leftheriotis G, Gomez-Merino D, et al. Effect of acute sleep deprivation on vascular function in healthy subjects. J Appl Physiol. 2010;108:68–75. https://doi.org/10.1152/japplphysiol.00851.2009.

61. Sekine T, Daimon M, Hasegawa R, et al. The impact of sleep deprivation on the coronary circulation. Int J Cardiol. 2010;144:266–7. https://doi.org/10.1016/j.ijcard.2009.01.013.

62. Kubo T, Fukuda S, Hirata K, et al. Comparison of coronary microcirculation in female nurses after day-time versus night-time shifts. Am J Cardiol. 2011;108:1665–8. https://doi.org/10.1016/j.amjcard.2011.07.028.

63. Plog BA, Nedergaard M. The glymphatic system in central nervous system health and disease: past, present, and future. Annu Rev Pathol. 2018;13:379–94. https://doi.org/10.1146/annurev-pathol-051217-111018.

64. Iliff JJ, Wang M, Liao Y, et al. A paravascular pathway facilitates CSF flow through the brain parenchyma and the clearance of interstitial solutes, including amyloid β. Sci Transl Med. 2012;4:147ra111. https://doi.org/10.1126/scitranslmed.3003748.

65. Mestre H, Tithof J, Du T, et al. Flow of cerebrospinal fluid is driven by arterial pulsations and is reduced in hypertension. Nat Commun. 2018;9:4878. https://doi.org/10.1038/s41467-018-07318-3.

66. Xie L, Kang H, Xu Q, et al. Sleep drives metabolite clearance from the adult brain. Science. 2013;342:373–7. https://doi.org/10.1126/science.1241224.

67. Plog BA, Dashnaw ML, Hitomi E, et al. Biomarkers of traumatic injury are transported from brain to blood via the glymphatic system. J Neurosci. 2015;35:518–26. https://doi.org/10.1523/JNEUROSCI.3742-14.2015.

68. Collins SD. Excess mortality from causes other than influenza and pneumonia during influenza epidemics. Public Heal Rep. 1932;47:2159. https://doi.org/10.2307/4580606.

69. Barnes M, Heywood AE, Mahimbo A, et al. Acute myocardial infarction and influenza: a meta-analysis of case-control studies. Heart. 2015;101:1738–47. https://doi.org/10.1136/heartjnl-2015-307691.

70. Warren-Gash C, Smeeth L, Hayward AC. Influenza as a trigger for acute myocardial infarction or death from cardiovascular disease: a systematic review. Lancet Infect Dis. 2009;9:601–10. https://doi.org/10.1016/S1473-3099(09)70233-6.

71. Kwong JC, Schwartz KL, Campitelli MA, et al. Acute myocardial infarction after laboratory-confirmed influenza infection. N Engl J Med. 2018;378:345–53. https://doi.org/10.1056/NEJMoa1702090.

72. Chiang M-H, Wu H-H, Shih C-J, et al. Association between influenza vaccination and reduced risks of major adverse cardiovascular events in elderly patients. Am Heart J. 2017;193:1–7. https://doi.org/10.1016/j.ahj.2017.07.020.

73. Nichol KL, Nordin J, Mullooly J, et al. Influenza vaccination and reduction in hospitalizations for cardiac disease and stroke among the elderly. N Engl J Med. 2003;348:1322–32. https://doi.org/10.1056/NEJMoa025028.

74. Davis MM, Taubert K, Benin AL, et al. Influenza vaccination as secondary prevention for cardiovascular disease: a science advisory from the American Heart Association/American College of Cardiology. Circulation. 2006;114:1549–53. https://doi.org/10.1161/CIRCULATIONAHA.106.178242.

75. Udell JA, Zawi R, Bhatt DL, et al. Association between influenza vaccination and cardiovascular outcomes in high-risk patients: a meta-analysis. JAMA. 2013;310:1711–20. https://doi.org/10.1001/jama.2013.279206.

76. Corrales-Medina VF, Alvarez KN, Weissfeld LA, et al. Association between hospitalization for pneumonia and subsequent risk of cardiovascular disease. JAMA. 2015;313:264–74. https://doi.org/10.1001/jama.2014.18229.

77. Cangemi R, Calvieri C, Falcone M, et al. Relation of cardiac complications in the early phase of community-acquired pneumonia to long-term mortality and cardiovascular events. Am J Cardiol. 2015;116:647–51. https://doi.org/10.1016/j.amjcard.2015.05.028.

78. Fountoulaki K, Tsiodras S, Polyzogopoulou E, et al. Beneficial effects of vaccination on cardiovascular events: myocardial infarction, stroke, heart failure. Cardiology. 2018;141:98–106. https://doi.org/10.1159/000493572.

79. Kang J-H, Ho J-D, Chen Y-H, Lin H-C. Increased risk of stroke after a herpes zoster attack: a population-based follow-up study. Stroke. 2009;40:3443–8. https://doi.org/10.1161/STROKEAHA.109.562017.

80. Minassian C, Thomas SL, Smeeth L, et al. Acute cardiovascular events after herpes zoster: a self-controlled case series analysis in vaccinated and unvaccinated older residents of the United States. PLoS Med. 2015;12:e1001919. https://doi.org/10.1371/journal.pmed.1001919.

81. Erskine N, Tran H, Levin L, et al. A systematic review and meta-analysis on herpes zoster and the risk of cardiac and cerebrovascular events. PLoS One. 2017;12:e0181565. https://doi.org/10.1371/journal.pone.0181565.

82. Hales CM, Harpaz R, Ortega-Sanchez I, et al. Update on recommendations for use of herpes zoster vaccine. MMWR Morb Mortal Wkly Rep. 2014;63:729–31.

83. Smith KR. Fuel combustion, air pollution exposure, and health: the situation in developing countries. Annu Rev Energy Environ. 1993;18:529–66. https://doi.org/10.1146/annurev.eg.18.110193.002525.

84. Clean Cooking Alliance. http://cleancookingalliance.org.

85. Klepeis NE, Nelson WC, Ott WR, et al. The National Human Activity Pattern Survey (NHAPS): a resource for assessing exposure to environmental pollutants. J Expo Anal Environ Epidemiol. 11:231–52. https://doi.org/10.1038/sj.jea.7500165.

86. Daigle CC, Chalupa DC, Gibb FR, et al. Ultrafine particle deposition in humans during rest and exercise. Inhal Toxicol. 2003;15:539–52. https://doi.org/10.1080/08958370304468.

87. Bräuner EV, Forchhammer L, Møller P, et al. Indoor particles affect vascular function in the aged: an air filtration-based intervention study. Am J Respir Crit Care Med. 2008;177:419–25. https://doi.org/10.1164/rccm.200704-632OC.

88. Allen RW, Carlsten C, Karlen B, et al. An air filter intervention study of endothelial function among healthy adults in a woodsmoke-impacted community. Am J Respir Crit Care Med. 2011;183:1222–30. https://doi.org/10.1164/rccm.201010-1572OC.

Index

© Springer Nature Switzerland AG 2019
A. Haverich and E. C. Boyle, *Atherosclerosis Pathogenesis and Microvascular Dysfunction*, https://doi.org/10.1007/978-3-030-20245-3

Printed in the United States
By Bookmasters